T0221107

Day Care
Anaesthesia

FUNDAMENTALS OF ANAESTHESIA AND ACUTE MEDICINE

Series editors

Ronald M Jones, Professor of Anaesthetics, St Mary's Hospital Medical School, London, UK
Alan R Aitkenhead, Professor of Anaesthetics, University of Nottingham, UK
Pierre Foëx, Nuffield Professor of Anaesthetics, University of Oxford, UK

Titles already available:

Anaesthesia for Obstetrics and Gynaecology
Edited by Robin Russell

Cardiovascular Physiology (second edition)
Edited by Hans Joachim Priebe and Karl Skarvan

Clinical Cardiovascular Medicine in Anaesthesia
Edited by Pierre Coriat

Intensive Care Medicine
Edited by Julian Bion

Management of Acute and Chronic Pain
Edited by Narinder Rawal

Neuro-Anaesthetic Practice
Edited by H Van Aken

Neuromuscular Transmission
Edited by Leo HDJ Booij

Paediatric Intensive Care
Edited by Alan Duncan

Forthcoming:

Day Care Anaesthesia
Edited by Ian Smith

Local and Regional Anaesthesia
Edited by Per H Rosenberg

Preoperative Assessment
Edited by Jeremy Cashman

Pharmacology of the Critically Ill
Edited by Maire Shelly and Gilbert Park

Fundamentals of Anaesthesia and Acute Medicine

Day Care Anaesthesia

Edited by
Ian Smith
Consultant Anaesthetist
North Staffordshire Hospital
Stoke-on-Trent

and

Senior Lecturer in Anaesthesia
Keele University
Staffordshire

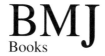

© BMJ Books 2000
BMJ Books is an imprint of the BMJ Publishing Group
www.bmjbooks.com

British Library Cataloguing in Publication Data
A catalogue record for this book is available from the
British Library

ISBN 0-7279-1422-7

Cover by Landmark Design, Croydon, Surrey
Typeset by Saxon Graphics Ltd, Derby
Printed and bound in Great Britain by MPG Books Ltd, Bodmin, Cornwall

Contents

To DA, Allison and Sam

Contributors

Angela Freschini, MB BS, FRCA
Specialist Registrar in Anaesthesia, North Staffordshire Hospital, Stoke-on-Trent, UK

Alexander P. L. Goodwin, FRCA
Consultant in Anaesthesia and Intensive Care, Lead Clinician for Day Surgery, Royal United Hospital NHS Trust, Bath, UK

Ian Jackson, FRCA
Director of Day Surgery Unit, York District Hospital, York, UK

Jan Jakobsson, MD PhD
Associate Professor, Department of Anaesthesia, Sabbatsberg Närsjuhuset, Sweden

Dori Ann McCulloch, MD
Consultant Anaesthetist, Staffordshire General Hospital, Stafford, UK

Jean M Millar, FRCA
Consultant Anaesthetist, Nuffield Department of Anaesthetics, Oxford, and Honorary Senior Clinical Lecturer, Medical School, Oxford University, Oxford, UK

John Peacock, FRCA
Consultant Anaesthetist, Royal Hallamshire Hospital, Sheffield, UK

Johan Ræder, MD, PhD
Professor of Anaesthesia, Chairman, Department of Anaesthesia, Ullevaal University Hospital, Oslo, Norway

Glenda Rudkin, MB, BS, FANZCA
Specialist Anaesthetist, Specialist Anaesthetic Services, Adelaide, Australia

Ian Smith, BSc MB BS, FRCA
Consultant Anaesthetist, North Staffordshire Hospital, Stoke-on-Trent, and Senior Lecturer in Anaesthesia, Keele University, Stoke-on-Trent, UK

Foreword

The Fundamentals of Anaesthesia and Acute Medicine series

The pace of change within the biological sciences continues to increase and nowhere is this more apparent than in the specialties of anaesthesia, acute medicine, and intensive care. Although many practitioners continue to rely on comprehensive but bulky texts for references, the accelerating rate of biomedical advances makes this source of information increasingly likely to be dated, even if the latest edition is used, The series *Fundamentals of Anaesthesia and Acute Medicine* aims to bring to the reader up-to-date and authoritative reviews of the principal clinical topics which make up the specialties. Each volume will cover the fundamentals or the topic in a comprehensive manner but will also emphasise recent developments of controversial issues.

International differences in the practice of anaesthesia and intensive care are now much less than in the past and the editors of each volume have commissioned chapters from acknowledged authorities throughout the world to assemble contributions of the highest possible calibre. Three volumes will appear annually and, as the pace and extent of clinically significant advances vary among the individual topics, new editions will be commissioned to ensure that practitioners will be in a position to keep abreast of the important developments within the specialties.

Not only does the pace of advance in biomedical science serve to justify the appearance of an international series of this nature but the current awareness of the need for more formal continuing education also underlines the timeliness of its appearances. The editors would welcome feedback from readers about the series, which is aimed at both established practitioners and trainees preparing for degrees and diplomas in anaesthesia and intensive care.

RONALD M JONES
ALAN R AITKENHEAD
PIERRE FOËX

Preface

The practice of day care surgery dates back more than 90 years, although it has only been over the last two decades that we have seen dramatic developments in this form of patient management. The recent expansion in day surgery began in the United States but a number of European and Australasian countries have seen similar growth in the subspecialty. Other countries are beginning to see the advantages of day surgery and have recently begun to, or are considering, expanding their programmes. Unquestionably, the major forces driving the expansion of day surgery are financial and political. The elimination of pre- and postoperative hospital admission, combined with a streamlined, efficient surgical procedure, significantly reduces direct costs. The separation of the need for surgery from the need for a hospital bed increases patient throughput and reduces waiting times, while releasing resources for other patient groups.

Despite these political and fiscal motives, day surgery turns out to be a good thing for patients! The need for careful preoperative evaluation, short-acting anaesthesia or sedation, and effective control of pain and nausea all ensure a high-quality experience for the patient. The high staffing ratios needed to cope with the rapid turnover of patients, combined with the need for active management during the recovery process, result in the patient feeling "cared for" and not sidelined as some "minor surgical patient" on a busy inpatient ward.

This book is intended as a convenient and practical guide for practitioners starting out in day surgery or trying to set up a day surgical unit. It will also be beneficial to established members of the team who may be expanding their practice, moving into different areas of work or who simply want to modify, update or improve their techniques. The authors have been selected from a number of countries in which day surgery is common. They are naturally experts in their field, with a wide background knowledge and familiarity with the latest drugs and techniques. More importantly, they were also chosen as practical, practising, hands-on day case anaesthetists. It was my intention, and I hope that I have achieved it, to encourage the authors to first provide a balanced overview of their subject and then descend from the fence and give their personal views or favourite techniques.

In a multiauthor book such as this, there will inevitably be a degree of overlap. Some I have removed but in other cases I have let the duplication remain to show where there is consistency of approach or difference of opinion. When experts are encouraged to state their preference, it will inevitably reveal different ways of achieving the same objectives; this will be especially apparent when comparing Chapters 3–6. The advice offered represents the opinion of the individual author. This will naturally represent a technique that works well for them, backed up by their considerable experience and, often, by a body of research evidence. Not everyone will find all the suggested techniques useful, while some will be controversial. However, I hope that this book will offer at least one practical solution to most problems that you, the reader, are likely to encounter. For the novice, this approach will make an excellent starting point to use while experience is gained or until a change proves necessary. For the more experienced, our suggestions may serve as an alternative for you to compare with your current practice.

A common theme running throughout this book is the need to follow up day case patients in order to audit and adapt practice. I strongly recommend that you adopt this approach, either when assessing the suggestions within this book or when using your own favourite techniques. This will ensure that your patients always receive the high-quality care that day surgery can, and should, provide.

Ian Smith

1: Patient selection, assessment, and preparation

Jean M Millar

Overview

This chapter is concerned with the selection of suitable procedures and patients for day case surgery. The importance of a variety of medical conditions will be discussed and guidance will be given on how these may be managed to ensure that the patient presents in optimum condition. A variety of methods of preoperative assessment will be introduced and the value of laboratory tests and other special investigations in preoperative evaluation will be reviewed.

Moving on from selection, the preoperative preparation of the day case patient will be considered, with regard to the management of chronic medication, preoperative fasting, and provision of information for patients and their carers. The subject of premedication will be discussed in its broadest sense to include the provision of analgesia, antiemesis, and aspiration prophylaxis as well as the relief of anxiety. The need for ongoing audit of perioperative problems in relation to selection criteria is stressed.

Introduction

The selection of suitable patients for suitable operations has long been regarded as the basis for good day surgical practice. However, the definition of "suitable" in this context has not always been based on clinical evidence but rather on the expectation that by excluding more major surgery and less fit patients, risks and complications might be eliminated. Recent practice has challenged these traditional views and procedures and patients previously considered inappropriate are now routinely undertaken on a day case basis. This is mainly due to economic pressures and shortage of inpatient beds but improvements in anaesthesia and pain control, minimally invasive surgical techniques and changing attitudes to recovery after surgery have all promoted the expansion of feasible day surgery patients and procedures.

Box 1.1 potential risks associated with day surgery

*Major risks**	*Minor risks***
Myocardial infarction	Minor anaesthetic complications
Pulmonary embolus	Pain
Respiratory failure	Nausea and vomiting (PONV)
Cerebrovascular accident	Dizziness, drowsiness
Major postoperative haemorrhage	Minor bleeding
Unrecognised damage to viscus	Infection
Major anaesthetic complications	Sore throat, headache

* Major risks have the potential for serious harm.

** Minor risks have little potential for serious harm.

From: Hitchcock M. Postoperative morbidity following day surgery. In: Millar JM, Rudkin GE, Hitchcock M, eds. *Practical anaesthesia and analgesia for day surgery*. Oxford: BIOS Scientific Publishers, 1997. With permission.

While every procedure carries some risk (Box 1.1), the incidence of major adverse events associated with day surgery is very low. Warner *et al.*[1] followed nearly 40 000 patients, 24% of whom were ASA 3, for 30 days after day surgery. There were only 31 cases (1:1455) of medically related major morbidity and mortality (myocardial infarction, pulmonary embolus, respiratory failure, and stroke), with two deaths from myocardial infarction. More than a third of these occurred more than 48 hours after surgery. This was similar to the risk for a similar population who had not had surgery. This low risk has been confirmed by other studies.[2–4]

Minor morbidity is much more common and has a lower potential for serious harm. However, it is important in the provision of a good service to patients and the smooth conduct of day surgery. These more minor problems have been related to some aspects of patient fitness but anaesthesia and surgery are generally more important, particularly in predicting unplanned overnight admission.[5–7] This makes setting strict criteria for patient selection both difficult and unhelpful. However, there is a need for some clear guidelines as to what is acceptable in terms of procedure and patient fitness, in the face of increasing pressure to carry out more invasive procedures on less fit patients.

Selection criteria

The Audit Commission's Day Surgery Report[8] in 1990 suggested a "basket" of common procedures that were considered suitable for day surgery (Box 1.2). While these are still valid, the extended use of minimally invasive techniques has increased the number of potential procedures and an expanded "trolley"[9] of procedures has been proposed by the British

Box 1.2 The Audit Commission's "basket" of suitable day case procedures, 1990. These procedures should be considered when establishing a day surgery programme

1. Inguinal hernia repair	11. Orchidopexy
2. Excision of breast lump	12. Cataract extraction±
3. Anal fissure excision	implant
4. Varicose vein stripping or ligation	13. Correction of squint
5. Cystoscopy, diagnostic and operative	14. Myringotomy ± grommets
6. Circumcision	15. Submucous resection
7. Excision of Dupuytren's contracture	16. Reduction of nasal fracture
8. Carpal tunnel decompression	17. Operation for bat ears
9. Athroscopy, diagnostic and operative	18. Dilatation and curettage
10. Excision of ganglion	19. Laparoscopy ± sterilisation
	20. Termination of pregnancy

From: reference[8]. With permission.

Association of Day Surgery (Box 1.3). Laparoscopic cholecystectomy is now routinely performed on a day case basis in some centres, as is tonsillectomy. In the United States, where the definition of ambulatory surgery encompasses a stay up to 23 hours and often extended recovery in specialised

Box 1.3 The British Association of Day Surgery's "trolley" of procedures, 1999. The Audit Commission's "basket" has been expanded to widen the range of procedures within the categories. Some other procedures were omitted as they were poor indicators of modern surgery

1. Groin/abdominal hernia repair (inguinal, femoral, umbilical, epigastric)	11. Inguinal surgery in children (orchidopexy and herniotomy)
2. Excision of breast lump	12. Cataract extract extraction ± implant
3. Minor anal surgery	
4. Varicose vein surgery	13. Correction of squint
5. Transurethral resection/diathermy/ laser of bladder tumours	14. Tonsillectomy in children
6. Circumcision (paediatric and adult)	15. Submucous resection
7. Release of Dupuytren's contracture	16. Reduction of nasal fractures
8. Carpal tunnel decompression	17. Bat ears/minor plastic procedures
9. Arthroscopy (incl. hip and shoulder)	18. Pilonidal sinus excision and closure
10. Hydrocele excision	19. Laparoscopy ± sterilisation
	20. Termination of pregnancy

Twenty further procedures where 50% should be possible as day cases are proposed:

1. Laparoscopic cholecystectomy
2. Laparoscopic herniorrhaphy
3. Thoracoscopic sympathectomy
4. Haemorrhoidectomy
5. Partial thyroidectomy
6. Submandibular gland excision
7. Superficial parotidectomy
8. Urethrotomy
9. Bladder neck incision
10. Laser prostatectomy
11. Transcervical resection of endometrium
12. Hallux valgus operations
13. Arthroscopic menisectomy
14. Arthroscopic shoulder surgery
15. Subcutaneous mastectomy
16. Wide excision of breast cancer with axillary clearance
17. Rhinoplasty
18. Eyelid surgery (incl. tarsorrhoplasty, blepharoplasty)
19. Tympanoplasty
20. Dentoalveolar surgery

From reference[9]. With permission.

centres, mastectomy, vaginal hysterectomy, thyroidectomy, laparoscopic Nissen fundoplication, shoulder stabilisations, and even radical retropubic prostatectomy and craniotomy have all been proposed as ambulatory procedures. This is driven by the health insurance companies and health maintenance organisations (HMOs) and has resulted in some backlash, with proposed legislation to prohibit the "drive-through" mastectomy. In general, however, intracranial, open abdominal, intrathoracic, and major vascular procedures are considered inappropriate because of the risk of serious postoperative sequelae and the need for close postoperative observation.

The principles of selection of suitable procedures are given in Box 1.4. Some of these are not clear cut.

- The risk of bleeding is a controversial issue. Paediatric tonsillectomy is routinely performed on a day case basis in many centres but anxiety about postdischarge bleeding deters others. However, the risk of serious primary haemorrhage can be virtually excluded if blood loss is small over an extended period of observation – 6–8 hours is usual.
- The duration of the procedure was previously considered important, with arbitrary limits of one or two hours, as morbidity and complications rise after this.[4, 6, 10] However, the invasiveness of the procedure rather than the duration is important. Laparoscopic surgery is associated with disproportionately increased morbidity and overnight admission, particularly for cholecystectomy.[6, 11, 12]

Box 1.4 Defining characteristics of appropriate day case procedures

- Minimal prolonged physiological trespass
- Not associated with excessive blood loss or fluid shifts
- Predictably stable postoperative course
- Minimal or no risk of serious postoperative complications, e.g.:
    bleeding
    thrombosis
    airway obstruction
    ileus
    electrolyte abnormalities
    seizures
    diminished level of consciousness
- Duration of 1–2 hours maximum?
- No need for surgical drains or urinary catheters?
- Oral intake feasible afterwards
- Pain controllable with oral/rectal analgesics after discharge
- Patient reasonably ambulant afterwards
- Predictable ability to discharge patient safely
- Appropriate staffing, equipment, and back-up for the procedure

- The pathology is important–small haemorrhoids or incisional hernias are suitable, very large ones may not be.
- The use of surgical drains has been considered a contraindication; if needed, these are usually removed before the patient goes home. Urinary catheters are surprisingly well tolerated and may allow urology patients to go home. Absorbable sutures and improved wound closure methods may reduce the need for patients to return for stitch removal.
- The day surgery facility must have the appropriate staffing, equipment, and back-up for the type of procedures being carried out. Free-standing or isolated sites need experienced personnel and a limited range of procedures.

Before introducing any more major operation as a day case procedure, it is imperative to have a "dry run" where the patients are treated as day cases but admitted overnight to monitor complications and problems. For more invasive operations, social and psychological factors should also be considered.

Suitable patients

Social factors

Patients must be discharged to safe and acceptable home conditions. This means there must be a responsible and physically able adult who can care for them at least overnight afterwards and longer for more invasive procedures. Elderly partners or several small children may make this difficult but if the question of postoperative care is discussed with the patient in good time, suitable arrangements can often be made.

For patient comfort and safety, travelling distance home should normally be less than one hour. Public transport should not be used and medical care must be reasonably accessible in case of complications. At home, there should be acceptable sanitary conditions, not too many stairs and access to a telephone. Nurses are usually much better than medical staff at identifying potential social problems and it is a useful part of the assessment visit.

Other options have been used where home circumstances are not ideal, such as hospital hotels supplying overnight supervision at low cost or, more rarely, transfer to a community hospital. An overnight stay in hospital (the "23 hour admit") may permit more procedures and patients to be "day cases", but may not achieve all the benefits of day surgery. Alternative social support is available in other countries and the "hospital at home" has been suggested: hospital-based nurses visit the patients in their own home afterwards. In the US, recovery centres may be used for patients who are unable to go home. There is clearly an increased cost in providing these options and they are generally not available in the UK.

Medical criteria

To the anaesthetist, good selection and preparation of day case patients are essential for minimising perioperative risk and allowing smooth uncomplicated treatment on the day. ASA (American Society of Anesthesiologists) status has not proved a very helpful predictive tool in this respect (except in the broadest sense), nor have arbitrary limits on age and weight. The low incidence of perioperative medical and anaesthetic complications in day cases makes identifying risk associated with specific medical conditions difficult. Also, within each group of patients with a specific medical problem, there is a spectrum of severity which needs to be evaluated.

In several large audits, adverse perioperative events in day surgery have been related to hypertension, severe symptomatic cardiac and respiratory disease, obesity, smoking, diabetes, and age [2, 4, 6, 10] (Box 1.5). Hypertension has been specifically related to intraoperative cardiovascular events, and asthma and smoking to postoperative respiratory events. Obesity (Body Mass Index [BMI] >30) relates to intraoperative and postoperative respiratory events[4]. Interestingly, the use of sedation increased intraoperative complications.[4, 10] Admission overnight is harder to attribute to patient fitness and the majority of cases are due to postoperative surgical and anaesthetic problems. The incidence of perioperative complications compared to that of similar patients having inpatient care has not been established, nor has a relationship with the need for overnight admission or later adverse

Box 1.5 Patient fitness and complications in day surgery

Perioperative complications have been found to be increased by:
- hypertension[2, 4, 10]
- symptomatic heart disease[10]
- symptomatic respiratory disease[2, 4, 10]
- obesity [2, 10]
- smoking [2, 10]
- diabetes[2]
- age >65[13]
- sedation [4, 10]

Unplanned overnight admission has been found to be increased by:

- longer surgery[5, 6, 10]
- type of surgery [5, 6]
- surgical complications[5]
- postoperative morbidity–pain, PONV [5, 6]
- age >65 [5, 6]
- ASA ≥2 [5, 6]

events. Would the same perioperative complications occur regardless of day or inpatient treatment? Where preoperative management or postoperative observation is not indicated, would admitting these patients before and/or after their operation change their clinical course?

Common principles for the care of all less fit patients for day surgery are:

- careful preadmission screening
- optimisation of their fitness before admission
- consideration of local or regional anaesthesia
- identification of the benefits of overnight admission pre- or postoperatively.

It is important that less fit patients are anaesthetised by experienced day surgery anaesthetists and not left to the more junior anaesthetic trainee.

Age

Age *per se* is not a contraindication to day surgery. It increases the likelihood of other diseases, especially hypertension and cardiac disease, so preoperative screening should be more careful in the over-70s. In a large prospective study, Chung *et al.* found that patients over 65 had a higher incidence of intraoperative events, particularly cardiovascular events, even when ASA status was corrected for, but had a lower incidence of postoperative pain, nausea, and dizziness.[13] They commented that this does not mean that age over 65 is a contraindication to day surgery but that older patients require more careful intraoperative cardiovascular management.

Many common procedures, such as cataract extraction, are well tolerated under local anaesthesia with minimal sedation and this may be an option for the less fit. However, postoperative confusion is common in the elderly, regardless of the type of anaesthesia or sedation,[14] and a period of observation is needed before discharge.

Social conditions should also be taken into consideration but in general, elderly patients benefit from returning to familiar surroundings, provided that there is sufficient home support.

Hypertension

Hypertension *is* important–it is one of the few identified predictors of perioperative myocardial ischaemia,[15] and complications and morbidity in day surgery.[2, 4, 10] Hypertensive patients should have their blood pressure (BP) controlled before any surgery and should not discontinue their medication.

Uncontrolled hypertension is probably the commonest cause of cancellation on the day of surgery and of acrimony from the surgeon and the general practitioner (GP), who finds the patient's BP to be within normal limits in his surgery. This "white coat" (or labile) hypertension has been shown to be a marker for underlying left ventricular disease[16] and elevated admission BP (>170/100) was a predictor of postoperative myocardial ischaemia.[17] However, these studies involved patients having more invasive surgery than is generally undertaken in day surgery, where the risk may be less. A reasonable BP for day surgery might be ≤175/105, although a hard and fast level is difficult to set.

Uncontrolled hypertension

How should we deal with the patient who presents unexpectedly on the day of surgery with an elevated BP? Clinical common sense suggests that other factors should then be considered. The anxious but otherwise fit woman, with no other risk factors, who is to have a potentially malignant breast lump removed is best treated by excision of the lump. The obese older male smoker, with a history of labile but untreated hypertension, for a hernia repair should have his BP controlled before surgery. A common misconception is that the problem may be solved by giving preoperative sedation: any anaesthetic or sedative drug will reduce the BP in the short term but will not deal with the underlying cardiac abnormalities or risk.

Hypertension identified at the screening clinic should be treated before surgery, ideally with β blockers.[18] A period of adjustment (typically 2–4 weeks) is needed before surgery as, in the short term, the use of β blockers is associated with intraoperative hypotension.[19] All hypertensive patients should have an ECG, as associated cardiovascular disease is common.

Cardiac disease

The severity of any cardiac disease needs to be assessed before admission. The American College of Cardiology/American Heart Association Task Force has provided excellent and comprehensive practice guidelines for the evaluation of patients for non-cardiac surgery.[20] These are to:

- identify the *presence* of cardiac disease
- define *severity*, *stability*, and any prior *treatment* needed
- evaluate other factors:
  - functional capacity (exercise tolerance)
  - other pathology: diabetes, peripheral vascular disease, renal failure, etc.
  - type of surgery.

In a day surgery population presenting for elective minor or intermediate procedures (by definition, lower risk surgery), most relevant cardiac-related symptoms can be detected at the routine preoperative assessment (see later). Exercise tolerance is a useful screening tool and can be calculated as metabolic equivalents (MET). Cardiac and long-term risk is increased in patients unable to meet a 4 MET demand.[21] This translates as climbing a flight of stairs. Risk factors are shown in Figure 1.1. Patients with major risk factors are unsuitable for day surgery. Exercise tolerance and the number of minor risk factors are what determine whether those at lower risk need further evaluation.

Asthma

Asthma is increasingly common, especially in younger patients. It is not a contraindication to day surgery, provided that the condition is well controlled and the patient has good exercise tolerance. Those who have required hospital admission or systemic steroids to control their asthma need more careful assessment and may need to be seen by the anaesthetist before admission if local anaesthesia is not an option. Peak expiratory flow and spirometry are more useful than a chest X-ray as they are better indicators of respiratory function. On the day, the patient's respiratory function should be optimal, without significant wheeze. The operation should be deferred if there is any upper or lower respiratory infection, which sensitises the airway and increases the chance of severe bronchospasm intraoperatively.

Non-steroidal antiinflammatory drugs (NSAIDs) trigger bronchospasm in around 5% of asthmatics. However, many asthmatic patients have taken aspirin or ibuprofen, the two over-the-counter NSAIDs, in the past without ill effect and in this case NSAIDs may be given for analgesia. All NSAIDs should be avoided in patients with known aspirin-sensitive asthma, as cross-reactivity is common.[22]

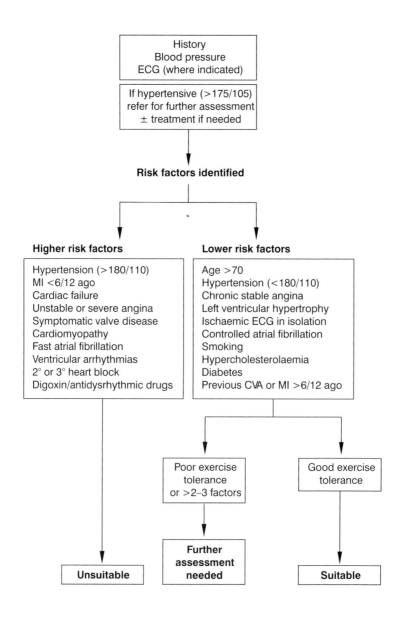

Figure 1.1 Cardiac evaluation of patients undergoing surgical procedures associated with low to moderate risk of perioperative ischaemia. ECG, electrocardiogram; MI, myocardial infarction; CVA, stroke or cerebrovascular accident. From: Millar JM. Selection and investigation of adult day cases. In: Millar JM, Rudkin GE, Hitchcock M, eds. *Practical anaesthesia and analgesia for day surgery*. Oxford: BIOS Scientific Publishers, 1997. With permission.

Chronic obstructive airways disease (COAD)
Unless patients with COAD are significantly restricted by their disease or have an acute exacerbation at the time of their surgery, they are suitable candidates. Again, exercise tolerance is the defining symptom triggering further investigation. Even patients with poor respiratory function may be able to have day surgery under local or regional anaesthesia, although sedation should be used with caution.

Acute upper respiratory tract infections (URTI)
These are unpredictable and patients presenting with colds on the day of surgery are a common winter problem. In adults with mild URTI, who are afebrile and have no signs of involvement of the lower respiratory tract, it is probably reasonable to proceed with surgery, unless it involves the airway.[23] Tracheal intubation should also be avoided, if at all possible.

Box 1.6 Problems which may be associated with obesity

The patient
Cardiovascular disease
Hypertension
Delayed gastric emptying, reflux, hiatus hernia
Diabetes
Sleep apnoea (especially if collar size >17 inches or 43 cm)

The anaesthetist
Lifting and handling
Venous access
Placing local anaesthetic blocks
Drug dosage calculations
Delayed recovery
Airway control and intubation
Hypoxaemia intra- and postoperatively

The surgeon
Increased surgical difficulty
Impossibility of some surgery, e.g. laparoscopy
Increased postoperative complications – deep vein thrombosis, wound breakdown, infection

---

Obesity
It is common practice in the UK (but not the US) to set limits for obesity in day surgery, because of increased problems for the patient, anaesthetist, and surgeon (Box 1.6). However, day surgery is less invasive, with minimal physiological trespass and postoperative morbidity, so the risk is considerably less than for more major surgery (Fig. 1.2). Laparoscopy and shared airway surgery occupy an intermediate position in this respect. Obviously if the patient is unfit and obese, and particularly if also a smoker, the risk will

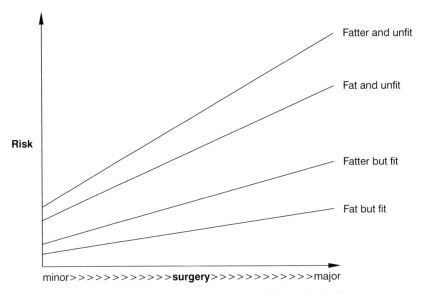

Figure 1.2 Risk versus procedure and fitness in obesity.

increase (Figure 1.2). Obesity *per se* has been related to intraoperative and immediate postoperative respiratory complications,[2,4,24] but not to overnight admission afterwards.[6,10]

Defining obesity
How is obesity measured? Body Mass Index (BMI; kg/m^2) is the commonest measurement used in the UK, with 30–35 being the usual limit (Box 1.7). However, in published studies, the degree of obesity is usually defined as BMI >30, with no differentiation for greater levels of obesity. There is a considerable difference between patients of BMI 30 and those of BMI >40 in the difficulty and hazards of anaesthesia and surgery. The most important parameter may be waist measurement as this relates to BMI, cardiovascular risk, and hypertension[25,26] and also to anaesthetic difficulties and postoperative hypoxaemia. Abdominal fat also makes surgery more difficult, particularly hernia repair and laparoscopy.

A personal audit of problems with obese day case patients having general anaesthesia has shown that perioperative problems, mainly mild hypoxaemia, become more apparent at BMI ≥37, with a steep increase once a value of 40 is reached. Despite more perioperative problems, there is no significant increase in overnight admission. This may be because day surgery anaesthesia is ideal for the obese patient, with rapid recovery and return of protective airway reflexes, and avoidance of the respiratory depressant effects of long-acting opioids. For peripheral procedures, the laryngeal mask airway gives good control of the airway and avoids the

Box 1.7 Measuring obesity

Body Mass Index (BMI) = kg/m^2

BMI <25	Normal
BMI 25–30	Overweight
BMI 30–35	Obese
BMI >35	Morbidly obese

Waist measurement & BMI[25]

BMI >30	>102 cm in men	>88 cm in women
BMI >35	>116 cm in men	>98 cm in women

hazards of intubation, which may be difficult, and associated with coughing and oxygen desaturation at extubation. If obese patients fulfil the usual discharge criteria there is no need to admit them overnight, unless there is a history of sleep apnoea.

The risk of gastrooesophageal reflux may not be as great as previously thought in the obese. Illing showed that obesity, laparoscopy, and a history of reflux did not increase intraoperative acid reflux but that this *was* associated with bucking and coughing on the endotracheal tube.[27] However, tracheal intubation is recommended for laparoscopic procedures in the very obese and in those with a history of hiatus hernia or postural reflux on lying down or bending. The use of H_2-receptor blockers and prokinetic agents may be helpful, particularly if these can be given before admission.

A sensible limit for day surgery *might* be BMI ≤35, although for more peripheral procedures, fatter patients are acceptable. Often no benefit can be identified from admitting these patients before or after surgery, as the problems are all related to the intraoperative and immediate postoperative period. Clearly careful preadmission assessment is needed to exclude those with significant systemic disease and sleep apnoea. Alternatives are the use of local or regional anaesthesia, although sedation should be used with caution. Advice to lose weight is seldom successful and in the very obese, the risks of any surgery should be weighed against the benefits.

Diabetes

Diabetes should not be underestimated. It is associated with cardiovascular disease, renal disease, and autonomic dysfunction and control may be suboptimal. Good preadmission assessment, including testing of blood sugar, creatinine, and electrolytes, and ECG in older patients, is essential.

Well-controlled non-insulin dependent patients (NIDDM) pose few problems in day surgery. Oral hypoglycaemic drugs should be omitted before surgery and blood sugar tested on the day before surgery.

Insulin-dependent diabetes (IDDM) increases perioperative adverse events, but not overnight admission.[2, 10] IDDM can be difficult to handle as

13

a day case. Even well-controlled IDDM patients can present on the day with abnormal blood sugars due to the unpredictable effects of stress and fasting. Their management is usually very labour intensive, although a regime called "moving the sun in the sky" has been described by Natof[28] (Box 1.8). Planned care is essential, often with the diabetologists. However, many IDDM patients are proficient at managing their own diabetes.

Box 1.8 The management of IDDM day surgery patients for general anaesthesia

---

Aim to return the patients as soon as possible to usual diet and environment

- Exclude young/brittle/ketotic diabetic patients
- The anaesthetist *must* assess the patient before admission
- Schedule as early as possible on day of surgery
- Omit morning insulin and breakfast and carry sugar in case of hypoglycaemia
- Test blood sugar on arrival and at least once during recovery
- Intravenous glucose infusion if required until ready to eat
- Choose technique to minimise PONV
- Resume normal regime as soon as possible after surgery, starting with the patient's usual morning insulin and breakfast even though it is later in the day   (= "moving the sun in the sky")
- Consider local or regional anaesthesia ± minimal sedation
- If no sedation is required, normal insulin and meals can be continued

---

From: Millar JM. Selection and investigation of adult day cases. In: Millar JM, Rudkin GE, Hitchcock M, eds. *Practical anaesthesia and analgesia for day surgery*. Oxford: BIOS Scientific Publishers, 1997. With permission.

In both NIDDM and IDDM, local anaesthesia may be used without fasting the patient or changing their diabetic regime and this may be the method of choice for suitable procedures.

Immunocompromised patients
Clearly the reason for the patient's immunocompromised status must be taken into account and relevant blood tests carried out. Overall, these patients benefit from avoiding hospital admission and its attendant risk of hospital-based infection.

Concomitant medications
Patients on certain drugs (e.g. systemic steroids, monoamine oxidase inhibitors, anticoagulants, digoxin, and antidysrhythmics) require individual evaluation in relation to the surgery and type of anaesthesia, as the condition for which the drugs are being taken is relevant, and the patient's management may be affected.

Monoamine oxidase inhibitors may need to be continued, as these drugs are often a last resort in severe depression. Pethidine must be avoided, but there are no adverse reactions to other opioids, such as fentanyl, alfentanil or morphine, or with general anaesthetics. Depending on the patient's mental state, local or regional blocks, with or without sedation, may be suitable. If needed, small doses of direct-acting vasopressors may be used.

Anticoagulants *must* be stopped and blood clotting levels checked on the day of surgery, which can cause delays. Where artificial heart valves are involved, communication with the cardiologist and/or haematologist may be needed to establish a safe clotting level. The need for heparin infusion precludes day surgery for these patients.

Oestrogen-containing contraceptives (OC) should only be stopped before operations on the lower limb, especially if a tourniquet is to be used. Four weeks is sufficient time and alternative contraception must be used. If not discontinued, subcutaneous low molecular weight heparin should be considered. The progesterone-only OC need not be stopped before any kind of surgery. (Combined oral contraceptives. *British National Formulary* 1999; 37:358). Oestrogen hormone replacement therapy (HRT) and surgery are more controversial; it is suggested that the need for stopping HRT before surgery be reviewed. (Hormone replacement therapy. *British National Formulary* 1999;37:323). However, in minor surgery not involving lower limbs and where early mobilisation is predicted, stopping HRT is unnecessary unless there are other risk factors such as obesity or a previous history of deep vein thrombosis or pulmonary embolus.

Preoperative investigations

Routine batteries of investigations are expensive and unnecessary for asymptomatic patients. They have not been shown to affect management [29,30] and are often ignored, even if they are abnormal.[31] The majority of abnormal results can be predicted from the patient's history.[29] A systematic review of the evidence of the value of routine preoperative testing[32] confirms that abnormal tests seldom change the patient's management and are poor at predicting adverse postoperative outcomes, but may have greater predictive power in defined high-risk populations. Selective and rational ordering of tests should be based on clinical assessment at the preoperative visit.[30] The introduction of an anaesthetist-led preoperative evaluation clinic at Stanford, USA, resulted in a 55% reduction in routine tests.[33]

Blood and urine tests

Full blood count (FBC), haemoglobin (Hb), platelet count and clotting studies
FBC and/or Hb are only indicated where a risk of anaemia might be expected from the patient's history (e.g. menorrhagia, rectal bleeding,

15

severe haematuria, renal disease) or proposed procedure. Perioperative risk in chronic anaemia does not rise until the Hb is ≤8 g/dl,[34] and no study of *routine* testing has found a patient with this level.[32] A significant level of chronic anaemia will result in dyspnoea, which will be apparent from the patient's history.

Similarly, routine white blood cell counts, platelet counts, and clotting screens should only be done where clinically indicated.

Sickle screening

Routine sickle screening may be omitted in *adults* with no history of haemolytic anaemia; it will only detect those with previously unidentified sickle cell trait, as the disease will have become apparent by adulthood. Also, defining those at risk of sickle cell disease is difficult because of ethnic mixing.[35]

Sickle trait does not affect management in day surgery procedures, where conditions which precipitate sickling (e.g. dehydration, hypoxaemia, hypotension, acidosis) are unlikely to occur with sufficient severity.[36] Even tourniquets have been suggested to be safe in sickle trait, provided the limb is exsanguinated first, which is generally routine practice.

Serum creatinine/urea, electrolytes and glucose

Significant disturbances of serum biochemistry in otherwise fit patients are extremely rare. Patients with renal disease or diabetes clearly need appropriate tests but they will be identified from the history. The need for electrolyte levels in patients on diuretic therapy is debatable – in some day surgery units this is not considered mandatory.

Urine testing

This has been recommended as a routine preoperative investigation[37] and at least has the merit of being cheap, although it does take up nursing time that could be better spent. The chance of picking up an unsuspected disease is very small.

Electrocardiogram (ECG)

Routine ECG has been recommended to detect previously unknown abnormalities, as well as to provide a baseline. However, abnormal ECGs in patients over 50 with no relevant symptoms, cardiac disease or risk factors are rare.[38] Identifying those patients with cardiac disease (previous myocardial infarction, angina, valvular heart disease) and risk factors (hypertension, peripheral vascular disease, diabetes or a past history of cardiac failure or cerebrovascular accident) accounts for the majority of abnormal ECGs.

There is an increased incidence of abnormal ECGs in older patients and those of worse ASA status, but the predictive power of preoperative ECGs for postoperative cardiac complications is poor.[32,39] Even in patients over 75, the chance of finding a previously undiagnosed infarct was <0.5%,[40] and it may still be difficult to determine the age of the infarct. Abnormal rhythms and fast atrial fibrillation will be diagnosed from the history and examination. Preoperative ECGs are indicated only for patients over 60, and those with cardiac disease and risk factors.[38]

Chest X-ray (CXR)

CXR is unnecessary for day surgery, as respiratory function tests yield more appropriate information. If the patient is thought to merit a CXR on clinical grounds, he or she is almost certainly unsuitable for anything other than minor surgery under local anaesthesia.

Appropriate investigations

From the foregoing discussion, it may be deduced that there is no place for routine investigations on asymptomatic patients for day surgery. All preoperative investigations should be determined by the individual patient's history and symptoms or by the procedure (e.g. Rhesus blood grouping before termination of pregnancy). It is more important to have an efficient screening process which detects those patients who need further investigation.

Assessment of adult day case patients

A simple but effective system of assessing day case patients is the goal. It is easy to pour resources into this without affecting outcome, so the objectives need to be clear. If these are met, the system should be cost effective.[41] The reduced workload for junior hospital doctors is an added benefit.

Objectives of preadmission assessment for day cases

- It should triage prospective patients into those who are fit, those who need further evaluation or treatment, and those who will need inpatient admission.
- It should reduce unnecessary investigations while targeting the patients who need them, with the results available on the day of surgery.
- It should enable more patients to be suitable for day surgery, by addressing problems such as high blood pressure or unsuitable home circumstances.

- It should reduce cancellation for predictable reasons on the day of surgery. Cancellations waste operating time and resources and, more importantly, distress the patient.
- It should speed up the process of admitting the patient on the day of surgery, when time is wasted assessing patients and chasing investigations, especially if this ultimately results in cancellation.
- By reducing the pressure to proceed with borderline patients, perioperative morbidity and unplanned overnight admission may be reduced. Although it is unwise to proceed with suboptimally prepared patients, there is inevitable pressure to do so on the day.
- The patient can be given information, any anxieties discussed, and the proposed date of surgery agreed. This improves compliance with pre- and postoperative instructions and reduces non-attendance. Patients are usually enthusiastic about assessment clinics even if it means an extra journey to hospital. They welcome the opportunity to ask questions in the more relaxed atmosphere of this setting.
- A potential benefit is the management of medicolegal risk. It is good practice to have a well-organised and documented assessment system.

Selection criteria

Clear selection criteria must be set out. These will inevitably vary according to the views of local anaesthetists and surgeons and the type of day care facility. Borderline patients may have to be assessed by the anaesthetist concerned if opinions on acceptable patients vary greatly. Freestanding units may restrict admission to fitter patients. If avoiding inpatient admission is a priority due to shortage of beds, operations and patients with a lower likelihood of admission may be selected.

Systems of patient assessment

The historical method has been for the surgeon to decide whether the patient is suitable for day surgery. However, most surgeons have neither the time to assess patients nor the appreciation of what constitutes fitness for anesthesia and surgeon assessment may be little better than no assessment at all.

The other end of the spectrum is the "anaesthesia preoperative evaluation clinic" developed in the USA.[33] In this model, every patient is seen by an anaesthetist, although not the one who will actually anaesthetise that patient. Although this is cost effective in the North American setting and has been shown to reduce preoperative investigations by 55% and costs by 59%[33], anaesthetists' time is scarce and expensive. It is unnecessary for every patient to see an anaesthetist during the initial screening process, but there must be anaesthetist back-up. Usually queries as to fitness for anaesthesia can be answered from the patient's history, with supplementary investigations if needed. The very occasional patient who does require it can be given an appointment to see an anaesthetist, preferably the one who will provide the anaesthesia. No benefits have been shown in the patient routinely meeting the anaesthetist before the day of surgery.[42]

You may be able to have your operation as a day case.
To help us plan your treatment, please answer the following questions.

Can an adult take you home by car or taxi after your operation? Yes ☐ No ☐
Is there a responsible and physically fit adult to look after you for
the first night after your operation? Yes ☐ No ☐
Would it take you less than
1 hour to get home from the hospital? Yes ☐ No ☐

Do you suffer from or have you ever suffered from:
Heart disease or a heart murmur Yes ☐ No ☐
High blood pressure Yes ☐ No ☐
Chest pains or angina Yes ☐ No ☐
Stroke Yes ☐ No ☐
Asthma Yes ☐ No ☐
Chronic cough or bronchitis Yes ☐ No ☐
Too breathless to climb 1 flight stairs Yes ☐ No ☐
Diabetes Yes ☐ No ☐
Epilepsy Yes ☐ No ☐
Kidney problems Yes ☐ No ☐
Bleeding problems Yes ☐ No ☐
Jaundice Yes ☐ No ☐
Heartburn or hiatus hernia Yes ☐ No ☐
Any other diseases Yes ☐ No ☐

If you answered YES to any of these questions, please tell us about it
....
....

Are you taking any tablets, pills, inhalers or medicine? Yes ☐ No ☐
If yes, please list them
....

Have you any allergies (including drug allergies)? Yes ☐ No ☐
If yes, please list them
....

Do you smoke? If YES, how many per day................. Yes ☐ No ☐
Do you have false, capped, crowned or loose teeth? Yes ☐ No ☐
Have you had any operations or anaesthetics before? Yes ☐ No ☐
If yes, please list
....

Were there any problems? If so please give details
....

Have any of your family had problems with anaesthetics? Yes ☐ No ☐

Figure 1.3 An example of an adult assessment questionnaire for day surgery. From Millar JM. Assessment and preparation of adult day cases. In Millar JM, Rudkin GE, Hitchcock M. eds. *Practical Anaesthesia and Analgesia for Day Surgery.* Oxford: BIOS Scientific Publishers, 1997. With permission.

DAY CARE ANAESTHESIA

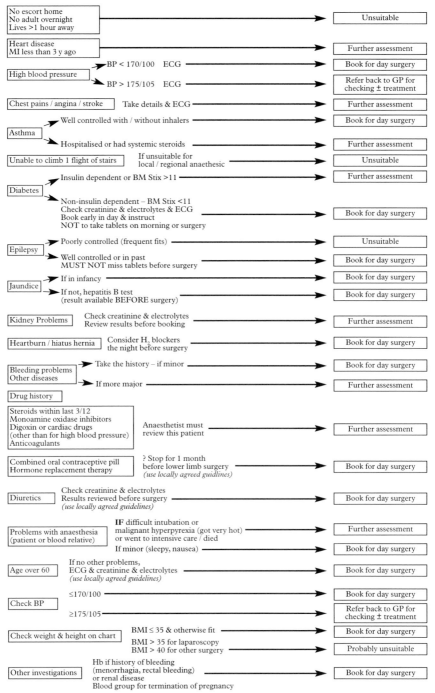

No escort home / No adult overnight / Lives >1 hour away	Unsuitable
Heart disease / MI less than 3 y ago	Further assessment
High blood pressure — BP < 170/100 ECG	Book for day surgery
High blood pressure — BP > 175/105 ECG	Refer back to GP for checking ± treatment
Chest pains / angina / stroke — Take details & ECG	Further assessment
Asthma — Well controlled with / without inhalers	Book for day surgery
Asthma — Hospitalised or had systemic steroids	Further assessment
Unable to climb 1 flight of stairs — If unsuitable for local / regional anaethesic	Unsuitable
Diabetes — Insulin dependent or BM Stix >11	Further assessment
Diabetes — Non-insulin dependent – BM Stix <11 / Check creatinine & electrolytes & ECG / Book early in day & instruct / NOT to take tablets on morning or surgery	Book for day surgery
Epilepsy — Poorly controlled (frequent fits)	Unsuitable
Epilepsy — Well controlled or in past / MUST NOT miss tablets before surgery	Book for day surgery
Jaundice — If in infancy	Book for day surgery
Jaundice — If not, hepatitis B test (result available BEFORE surgery)	Book for day surgery
Kidney Problems — Check creatinine & electrolytes / Review results before booking	Further assessment
Heartburn / hiatus hernia — Consider H₂ blockers the night before surgery	Book for day surgery
Bleeding problems / Other diseases — Take the history – if minor	Book for day surgery
Bleeding problems / Other diseases — If more major	Further assessment
Drug history	
Steroids within last 3/12 / Monoamine oxidase inhibitors / Digoxin or cardiac drugs (other than for high blood pressure) / Anticoagulants — Anaesthetist must review this patient	Further assessment
Combined oral contraceptive pill / Hormone replacement therapy — ? Stop for 1 month before lower limb surgery (use locally agreed guidlines)	Book for day surgery
Diuretics — Check creatinine & electrolytes / Results reviewed before surgery (use locally agreed guidelines)	Book for day surgery
Problems with anaesthesia (patient or blood relative) — IF difficult intubation or malignant hyperpyrexia (got very hot) or went to intensive care / died	Further assessment
Problems with anaesthesia — If minor (sleepy, nausea)	Book for day surgery
Age over 60 — If no other problems, ECG & creatinine & electrolytes (use locally agreed guidelines)	Book for day surgery
Check BP — ≤170/100	Book for day surgery
Check BP — ≥175/105	Refer back to GP for checking ± treatment
Check weight & height on chart — BMI ≤ 35 & otherwise fit	Book for day surgery
Check weight & height on chart — BMI > 35 for laparoscopy / BMI > 40 for other surgery	Probably unsuitable
Other investigations — Hb if history of bleeding (menorrhagia, rectal bleeding) or renal disease / Blood group for termination of pregnancy	Book for day surgery

Patients who are unsuitable for general anaesthesia may be able to have local anaesthesia as a day case
Request anaesthetic opinion if in doubt

The best system is for trained nurses to undertake the screening with the help of patient questionnaires (Fig. 1.3) and a structured protocol detailing action to be taken (Fig. 1.4). In some centres,[43] the questionnaire is completed by the patient in the surgical outpatient clinic and evaluated later by nurses in the day unit. This system avoids the need for an additional patient visit and appears to work well.[43] More commonly, the patient attends a nurse-led clinic, where checks on height, weight, and blood pressure are also included. Computer systems are now available to assist with this. Nurse-led clinics have been shown to reduce cancellations and doctors' workload.[44] In addition, nurses are arguably better than doctors at recognising problems with home background and at taking time to discuss the patients' queries and anxieties. The timing of the assessment visit should be far enough ahead to allow any problems to be sorted out, but not so far in advance that the patient's health has deteriorated before admission. Two to four weeks before surgery is probably optimal. Having some evening clinics avoids patients taking time off work.

Rigid selection criteria with no anaesthetic referral system will lead to many suitable day case patients being turned away. It is essential to have an identified anaesthetist to provide leadership for the assessment clinic and support for the nurses.

GPs may become involved in assessment, as they have access to the information which is needed. A similar system of providing them with a protocol and anaesthetic back-up would be needed. Another option is telephone screening which works well for younger, fitter patients, who may be spared a journey. This works better if the patient is asked to telephone the clinic and evening sessions may be needed for this. If needed, investigations and BP can be arranged with the GP and borderline cases can be asked to attend for further assessment.

When should the anaesthetist meet the patient?

Meeting the anaesthetist before admission is rarely necessary and does not reduce anxiety or increase patient satisfaction, compared to meeting him or her on the day of admission.[42] The Royal College of Anaesthetists' guidance on day case anaesthesia[45] states that the anaesthetist must have an opportunity to talk to the patient before the procedure on the day of operation, so that rapport can be established and any last minute questions addressed. It is unacceptable for the anaesthetist to encounter the patient for the first time in the anaesthetic room or operating theatre, even if fit, healthy, and well screened. Time must be allowed for this visit, despite pressure from surgeons and managers.

Figure 1.4 (facing page) Assessment guidelines for patients having general anaesthesia. MI, myocardial infarct; BP, blood pressure; ECG, electrocardiogram; BM stix, finger prick blood sugar test; BMI, body Mass Index. From Millar JM. Assessment and preparation of adult study cases. In Millar JM Rudkin GE, Hitchcock M, eds. *Practical anaesthesia and analgesia for day surgery.* Oxford: BIOS Scientific Publishers, 1997. With permission.

21

Preparation of the patient

Part of the screening process is to prepare the patient for surgery. Good preparation and information improve compliance and reduce cancellations for reasons other than physical fitness (Box 1.9). In particular, discussing the patient's concerns, agreeing a date for the operation, and verifying care at home are likely to be beneficial in reducing cancellations and non-attenders. If local or regional anaesthesia (with or without sedation) is an option, nursing protocols will be needed to identify appropriate patients.

Box 1.9 Reasons for postponed or cancelled operations unrelated to physical fitness

---

- Inability to keep the appointment
- Fear or anxiety about the procedure
- Patient decides not to proceed with surgery
- Change in the surgical condition
- Failure to arrange escort or overnight supervision
- Failure to make suitable arrangements for time off work or child care
- Failure to comply with fasting instructions
- Failure to comply with instructions for medication
- Failure to notify the day surgery unit of acute medical conditions

---

From: Millar JM. Selection and investigation of adult day cases. In: Millar JM, Rudkin GE, Hitchcock M, eds. *Practical anaesthesia and analgesia for day surgery.* Oxford: BIOS Scientific Publishers, 1997. With permission.

Fasting instructions

It is now generally agreed that prolonged fluid fasts are unnecessary and increase patient discomfort. The ASA Task Force on Preoperative Fasting has produced practice guidelines for healthy patients for elective surgery. Solids and milk should still be stopped six hours before surgery (and meat and fried food eight hours before), but clear fluids may be taken up to two hours before surgery.[46] The volume is less important than the type of fluid:free clear fluids up to two hours before the procedure do not affect gastric volume or pH.[47] Unless the time of operation is predictable, scheduling oral fluids may be difficult but a reasonable plan is to allow a drink 1–2 hours before admission, followed by more later after arrival if the wait is likely to be more than two hours.

Medication

Regular medication, such as antihypertensive, anticonvulsant, steroid or bronchodilator drugs, should be taken as usual before surgery. The only exceptions to this generalisation are oral hypoglycaemics, insulin, anticoagulants, and oestrogen-containing oral contraceptives. Some of these patients will need reviewing by the anaesthetist before admission to plan their care.

Restrictions on postoperative activity

Patients need to know what they may not do after their surgery. This includes the period for which they should not drive or operate machinery and time of returning to work, which will be dependent on the operation.

Preadmission information

Clear written instructions are needed to back up information given verbally. Important items should be succinct and all on the front page as, bombarded by information, the patient may read none of it. Separate booklets or leaflets about what will happen on the day and during the procedure itself can be given at the time of screening or sent to the patient. Suggestions for the content of the information are given in Box 1.10.

Producing good information for patients is not as easy as it sounds. Guidelines for information sheets are suggested in Box 1.11. Using computers to produce them means that information can be regularly updated easily. Tapes and videos may also be used. Reviews of whether patients read, understand, and approve of these educational materials should be carried out.

Premedication

Premedication is frequently omitted in day surgery in the belief that it is unnecessary and that sedative premedication delays recovery. In this context, premedication refers to drugs given *before* the patient arrives in the operating suite, rather than drugs administered intravenously at or just before induction of anaesthesia, which is co-induction.

There are practical problems which discourage the use of premedication. There may be insufficient time after the patient's arrival for drugs to be effective by the time of anaesthesia and surgery. In practice, premedication needs to be given orally or rectally, as the intravenous route causes logistical problems of administration and monitoring. The use of sedative drugs may also mean that the patient needs supervision and is unable to walk to the operating theatre suite.

Has preoperative medication therefore any place in day surgery and are there any benefits to be gained from it? The possible indications for premedication are given in Box 1.12.

Box 1.10 Preadmission information

On the front–important information
- Time and date of the operation
- The need for an escort and taxi or car to go home (not public transport)
- Instructions not to drive or operate machinery for 24–48 hours
- Fasting instructions
- Do not omit medication unless specifically requested to do so
- Instructions for clothing, valuables, and something to pass the time
- Contact telephone number if unable or unfit to keep the appointment
- For women, ring the day surgery unit if there is a possibility that you might be pregnant

Other information on the DSU and what will happen on the day
- Map, parking and how to find the day surgery unit
- Nursing procedures before surgery
- Anaesthetic assessment: pain, PONV, anxiety, and needle phobia
- Surgical: last minute questions and consent if not already signed
- Description of the trip to the operating theatre and the recovery process
- Duration of stay and time for escort to come
- Postanaesthetic restrictions on driving, alcohol, taking decisions, etc.
- Who to contact after discharge and follow-up arrangements

Procedure-specific information
- What the operation is, in simple non-frightening terms ± diagrams/pictures
- Preoperative preparation, e.g. shaving
- Time required off work and resuming normal activities
- Expected postoperative morbidity
- When to seek advice–postoperative problems
- Wound management, stitch removal, and follow-up if relevant

---

From: Millar JM. Assessment and preparation of adult day cases. In: Millar JM, Rudkin GE, Hitchcock M, eds. *Practical anaesthesia and analgesia for day surgery.* Oxford: BIOS Scientific Publishers, 1997. With permission.

Anxiolysis and sedation

It is generally believed that day case patients are not anxious and that giving anxiolytic drugs delays their recovery and discharge. However, many patients are very anxious, particularly young patients or those about to undergo certain types of surgery–especially breast lumpectomy, oral surgery or circumcision. Anxiety tends to increase between admission and arrival in the operating theatre and the use of intravenous drugs at induction does not reduce this. Studies have found that two-thirds of patients would like sedative premedication,[48] and that the majority of patients felt that they had benefited from it.[49]

Good day surgery practice can also reduce much of this anxiety (Box 1.13). The extremely anxious patient can be identified at assessment or at the preoperative anaesthetic visit on the day of surgery. Often a sympathetic

Box 1.11 Do's and don'ts of written patient information

- Give all instructions in written form (as well as verbal where possible)
- Have versions available in appropriate languages
- Keep them simple, succinct, and to the point or patients may not read any of them
- Use short sentences with active verbs and clear expressions
- Use a friendly style but do not patronise
- Avoid medical jargon, e.g. sublingual should be replaced with 'under your tongue'
- Do not use slang words for body parts
- Avoid jokes–they may not be funny to the patient
- Be positive–say what should be done
- Consider including "questions that patients often ask about their surgery"
- Coordinate procedure information with individual surgeons' practice
- Layout and style should be attractive and easy to read, with bold headings
- Put all the important points briefly on the front page
- Make sure a contact telephone number is prominently displayed
- Computers make information easy and cheap to update and personalise
- Assess whether patients read, understand, and approve of the information
- Edit and review regularly

From: Millar JM. Assessment and preparation of adult day cases. In: Millar JM, Rudkin GE, Hitchcock M, eds. *Practical anaesthesia and analgesia for day surgery*. Oxford: BIOS Scientific Publishers, 1997. With permission.

Box 1.12 Possible indications for premedication in day surgery

- Anxiolysis and sedation
- Reduction of risk factors for acid reflux and aspiration
- Antiemesis
- Analgesia–venepuncture and postoperative
- Other drugs–e.g. asthma prophylaxis

From: Millar JM. Premedication in adult day surgery. In: Millar JM, Rudkin GE, Hitchcock M, eds. *Practical anaesthesia and analgesia for day surgery*. Oxford: BIOS Scientific Publishers, 1997. With permission.

Box 1.13 Non-pharmacological measures to relieve anxiety

- Preoperative visit to the day surgery facility
- Good information on the whole of the surgical episode:
  - preparation before coming in
  - what can be expected on the day
  - recovery afterwards, including limitations on work and other activities
- Taking time to listen to the patient's concerns
- Reassurance from anaesthetist and nursing staff on the day

approach and the offer of premedication (if needed) is sufficient for many patients, who may then choose not to take sedative medication. However, some very anxious patients may need an anxiolytic drug at home before coming in.

Choice of anxiolytic

If anxiolysis is needed, what drugs are suitable? Achieving a balance between effective preoperative relief of anxiety and lack of postoperative hangover effects requires a careful choice of agent and dose. Short-acting benzodiazepines, usually midazolam or temazepam, are the most commonly used. Although midazolam is the more anxiolytic drug, it is also associated with a greater delay in recovery[48, 49] and its amnesic properties may interfere with postoperative recall of instructions.[50] Midazolam 7.5 mg orally was less effective at reducing anxiety than 15 mg, but still delayed psychomotor recovery.[51] Temazepam 10 mg or 20 mg orally have both been shown to reduce anxiety; the larger dose is better at reducing anxiety but delays immediate (but not later) recovery more than the lower dose.[52, 53]

Flumazenil has been suggested as an option to reverse the effects of benzodiazepines. After intravenous midazolam, it is temporarily effective but resedation is a danger.[54] The use of flumazenil has not been reported after oral benzodiazepines.

Other drugs suggested for sedation and anxiolysis in day surgery have included:

- *propofol*, used in patient-controlled devices, but the difficulties in setting these up and monitoring effects preclude their wide acceptance
- *opioids* in the form of sufentanil nasal sprays or fentanyl "lollipops", which provide less anxiolysis and are usually associated with increased nausea and vomiting
- *β-blocking drugs* (e.g. propranolol 80 mg orally or timolol 10 mg orally), which are effective but may cause intraoperative hypotension
- *α-adrenergic agonists* (e.g. clonidine and dexmetomidine), which cause prolonged sedation and are best avoided.

As a general recommendation for adults who need sedative premedication, midazolam 7.5 mg or, preferably, temazepam 10–20 mg 30–60 minutes before anaesthesia may be given orally.

Acid reflux and aspiration

Although the incidence of gastric reflux is rare (and that of aspiration even rarer) in day cases, there are theoretically many potential factors in day surgery predisposing to increased risk (Box 1.14). Risk is frequently defined as gastric contents ≥ 25 ml and pH ≤ 2.5, although there is now much doubt as to the validity of these figures in humans. Many of the potential risk factors are now also disputed. Anxiety, obesity, laparoscopy, and even symptomatic reflux were not shown to increase the risk of intraoperative acid reflux.[27] No significant increase in risk factors was shown in day case patients compared with inpatients, but 48% of day cases and 40% of inpatients had both "risk factors" of increased gastric volume and low pH.[55] Such evidence has been used as an argument for the use of prophylaxis in all patients, particularly if endotracheal intubation is not to be used. However, the "risk factors" occur with enormously greater frequency than actual aspiration and neither the face-mask nor the laryngeal mask have been demonstrated to increase the incidence of regurgitation in comparison to tracheal intubation. In contrast, coughing and bucking on an endotracheal tube have been associated with acid regurgitation.[27] Allowing clear fluids up to 2–3 hours preoperatively may actually have a beneficial effect in reducing the volume and acidity of stomach contents.

Box 1.14 Possible risk factors for gastric reflux in ambulatory patients

- Fasting instructions for solids disobeyed
- Anxiety
- Obesity
- Diabetes
- Early pregnancy
- Hiatus hernia or symptomatic gastric reflux
- Laparoscopic procedures

From: Millar JM. Premedication in adult day surgery. In: Millar JM, Rudkin GE, Hitchcock M, eds. *Practical anaesthesia and analgesia for day surgery* Oxford: BIOS Scientific Publishers, 1997. With permission.

Prophylaxis against reflux

H_2 receptor antagonists are the best drugs to increase gastric pH. Orally administered ranitidine (150 mg) is very effective, more so than sodium citrate,[56] cimetidine,[57] famotidine or omeprazole.[58] One hour is usually adequate for ranitidine to be effective, although a longer interval may make it even more effective. For high-risk patients, 150–300 mg given the night before and on arrival may further reduce risk.

H_2-receptor antagonists do not reliably reduce gastric volume but the addition of a prokinetic agent such as metoclopramide 10 mg orally may help to empty the stomach and increase lower oesophageal barrier pressure. Adverse effects are rare and the cost of these drugs given orally is cheap; it is difficult to justify the use of more expensive drugs such as omeprazole when this combination has been shown so convincingly to be effective at lowering gastric volume and acidity.

The ASA Task Force on Preoperative Fasting[46] also considered the use of drugs to reduce the risk of pulmonary aspiration and concluded that, while prokinetic agents, H_2-receptor antagonists, and proton pump inhibitors are effective in reducing acidity and volume, their routine use is not recommended, although the Task Force and their consultant advisors were equivocal about their use. It should be noted that many UK day units use no form of routine aspiration prophylaxis without any apparent increase in the incidence of pulmonary aspiration.

Antiemetic prophylaxis

Antiemetic drugs are usually administered intravenously during the procedure if their prophylactic use is considered necessary. Those with undesirable side effects such as sedation and dry mouth should be avoided (e.g. scopolamine patches, antihistamines, and anticholinergics). Preoperative droperidol can cause restlessness and dysphoria. The use of ranitidine and metoclopramide may contribute to reducing PONV, although metoclopramide's efficacy as an antiemetic has been questioned. The use of antiemetic medication is discussed further in Chapter 7.

Prophylactic analgesia

Non-steroidal antiinflammatory drugs (NSAIDs) have gained well-deserved popularity in day surgery because they reduce or eliminate the need for opioid analgesics which are associated with unacceptable side effects. It may be advantageous as well as economical to give NSAIDs orally as premedication,[59, 60] as this allows time for them to be effective when the patient wakes, particularly if the procedure is short, so avoiding the need to give opioids for rescue analgesia in the recovery room. Even given intravenously, NSAIDs take at least 30 minutes to work and parenteral preparations are generally more expensive than their oral equivalents. In practice, larger loading doses of simple and cheap NSAIDs such as ibuprofen 600–800 mg or diclofenac 100 mg by mouth one hour preoperatively are as (or more) effective as giving NSAIDs during surgery when the operating time is short. There is no evidence that expensive NSAIDs such as ketorolac are any more effective than ibuprofen or diclofenac, which are cheaper, longer lasting and have fewer adverse effects.

Enteric-coated preparations are absorbed from the duodenum, so giving a prokinetic drug such metoclopramide may help speed up absorption if more expensive soluble preparations are not used. Long-acting NSAID formulations, designed for slow release, may not achieve a sufficiently high serum level fast enough. However, slow-release ibuprofen 1600 mg (the recommended daily dose) appears to provide effective and long-lasting analgesia in practice, although there have been few objective studies conducted. The use of an H_2 antagonist will mitigate the effect of NSAIDs on an empty stomach, although single doses appear well tolerated by most patients in practice. Slow-release preparations may be even better in this regard.

Rectal NSAIDs are popular given during or after surgery and their use as premedication has been advocated. However, there is no intrinsic advantage to the rectal route and many patients are reluctant to self-administer suppositories.

NSAIDs should probably not be given before procedures such as tonsillectomy or laser prostatectomy, where they may increase blood loss. In operations associated with blood loss, NSAIDs may be given when the risk of bleeding is reduced. The use of prophylactic analgesia and the NSAIDs is further discussed in Chapter 7.

Analgesia for venepuncture
Even adults may be anxious about venepuncture and a sympathetic preoperative visit will detect this. EMLA® (lignocaine 2.5% and prilocaine 2.5% in a eutectic mixture) 60 minutes preoperatively or amethocaine 4% gel (Ametop®) 35–40 minutes preoperatively are effective in adults, although not perhaps quite as much as in children. An inhalation induction with sevoflurane (see Chapter 3) may be a preferable alternative for some needle phobics.

Other preoperative medication
The need for administration of other drugs is no different from inpatient surgery; for example, extra doses of bronchodilators in asthmatic patients, antibiotics before urological procedures and prostaglandins to facilitate termination of pregnancy may be required.

Effectiveness of patient selection, assessment, and preparation

In order to establish how well the system is working, non-attendance, cancellations, adverse events, and unplanned admissions should be regularly reviewed. Any problems which are identified should be addressed promptly. The reasons for rejecting patients for day surgery should also be reviewed to ensure that selection criteria are not too rigid, thereby excluding suitable patients. In the current climate of bed shortages, many patients will wait a long time for inpatient treatment. Patients should be asked whether they found the assessment process reassuring and informative or time consuming and inconvenient, and for more general views on their preoperative management.

Summary

Patient selection, assessment, and preparation for day surgery is a collaborative process involving the surgeon, anaesthetist, nursing staff, and patient. Teamworking is essential and anaesthetic input is imperative. Careful assessment is important and can best be accomplished with a well-designed questionnaire and a nurse-led screening process. Routine preoperative testing adds nothing of value, but clinically directed tests are important.

Once screened, patients with preexisting diseases may require further management to ensure their condition is optimal. There are no cast iron contraindications to day surgery, except an unwilling patient, and a flexible attitude backed up with common sense is what is needed.

Before surgery, patients should be adequately prepared with appropriate information. Premedication may occasionally be useful to reduce anxiety, protect at-risk patients against aspiration, and prevent postoperative nausea. For most patients, prophylactic provision of analgesia, combined with kindness and comprehensible explanation, may be all that are required. As with other areas of day case practice, preoperative procedures should be audited regularly and modified if necessary.

1   Warner MA, Shields SE, Chute CG. Major morbidity and mortality within 1 month of ambulatory surgery and anesthesia. *JAMA* 1993;**270**:1437–41.
2   Duncan PG, Cohen MM, Tweed WA *et al.* The Canadian four-centre study of anaesthetic outcomes: III. Are anaesthetic complications predictable in day surgical practice? *Can J Anaesth* 1992;**39**:440–8.
3   Natof HE. Complications associated with ambulatory surgery. *JAMA* 1980;**244**:1116–18.
4   Chung F, Mezei G, Tong D. Pre-existing medical conditions as predictors of adverse events in day-case surgery. *Br J Anaesth* 1999;**83**:262–70.
5   Fortier J, Chung F, Su J. Unanticipated admission after ambulatory surgery–a prospective study. *Can J Anaesth* 1998;**45**:612–19.
6   Gold BS, Kitz DS, Lecky JH, Neuhaus JM. Unanticipated admission to the hospital following ambulatory surgery. *JAMA* 1989;**262**:3008–10.
7   Paix A, Rudkin GE, Osborne GA. Ambulatory surgery complications and patient fitness. *Amb Surg* 1994;**2**:166–70.
8   Audit Commission. *A short cut to better services. Day surgery in England and Wales*. London: HMSO, 1990.
9   Cahill CJ. Basket cases and trolleys. Day surgery proposals for the Millennium. *J One-day Surg* 1999;**9**(1):11–12.
10   FASA. Special study 1. 700 N. Fairfax Street, No 520, Alexandria, Virginia 221314: 1986.
11   Tuckey JP, Morris GN, Peden CJ, Tate JJ. Feasibility of day case laparoscopic cholecystectomy in unselected patients. *Anaesthesia* 1996;**51**:965–8.
12   Singleton RJ, Rudkin GE, Osborne GA, Watkins DS, Williams JAR. Laparoscopic cholecystectomy as a day surgery procedure. *Anaesth Intens Care* 1996;**24**:231–6.
13   Chung F, Mezei G, Tong D. Adverse events in ambulatory surgery. A comparison between elderly and younger patients. *Can J Anaesth* 1999;**46**:309–21.
14   Chung F, Meier R, Lautenschlager E, Carmichael FJ, Chung A. General or spinal anesthesia: which is better in the elderly? *Anesthesiology* 1987;**67**:422–7.
15   Howell SJ, Hemming AE, Allman KG, Glover L, Sear JW, Foëx P. Predictors of postoperative myocardial ischaemia. The role of intercurrent arterial hypertension and other cardiovascular risk factors. *Anaesthesia* 1997;**52**:107–11.
16   Glen SK, Elliott HL, Curzio JL, Lees KR, Reid JL. White-coat hypertension as a cause of cardiovascular dysfunction. *Lancet* 1996;**348**:654–7.
17   Allman KG, Muir A, Howell SJ, Hemming AE, Sear JW, Foëx P. Resistant hypertension and preoperative silent myocardial ischaemia in surgical patients. *Br J Anaesth* 1994;**73**:574–8.
18   Stone JG, Foëx P, Sear JW, Johnson LL, Khambatta HJ, Triner L. Risk of myocardial ischaemia during anaesthesia in treated and untreated hypertensive patients. *Br J Anaesth* 1988;**61**:675–9.

19 Stone JG, Foëx P, Sear JW, Johnson LL, Khambatta HJ, Triner L. Myocardial ischemia in untreated hypertensive patients: effect of a single small dose of a beta-adrenergic blocking agent. *Anesthesiology* 1988;**68**:495–500.

20 Eagle KA, Brundage BH, Chaitman BR *et al.* Guidelines for perioperative cardiovascular evaluation for noncardiac surgery. Report of the American College of Cardiology/ American Heart Association Task Force on Practice Guidelines. Committee on Perioperative Cardiovascular Evaluation for Noncardiac Surgery. *Circulation* 1996;**93**:1278–317.

21 Fletcher GF, Balady G, Froelicher VF, Hartley LH, Haskell WL, Pollock ML. Exercise standards. A statement for healthcare professionals from the American Heart Association Writing Group. *Circulation* 1995;**91**:580–615.

22 Power I. Aspirin-induced asthma (editorial). *Br J Anaesth* 1993;**71**:619–21.

23 Fennelly ME, Hall GM. Anaesthesia and upper respiratory tract infection–a non-existent hazard (editorial)? *Br J Anaesth* 1990;**64**:535–6.

24 Rose DK, Cohen MM, Wigglesworth DF, DeBoer DP. Critical respiratory events in the postanesthesia care unit. Patient, surgical, and anesthetic factors. *Anesthesiology* 1994;**81**:410–18.

25 Lean ME, Han TS, Morrison CE. Waist circumference as a measure for indicating need for weight management. *Br Med J* 1995;**311**:158–61.

26 Han TS, van Leer EM, Seidell JC, Lean ME. Waist circumference action levels in the identification of cardiovascular risk factors: prevalence study in a random sample. *Br Med J* 1995;**311**:1401–5.

27 Illing L, Duncan PG, Yip R. Gastroesophageal reflux during anesthesia. *Can J Anaesth* 1992;**39**:466–70.

28 Natof H. Complications. In: Wetchler BV, ed. *Anesthesia for ambulatory surgery*, 2nd edn. Philadelphia: JB Lippincott, 1990.

29 Johnson H Jr, Knee-Ioli S, Butler TA, Munoz E, Wise L. Are routine preoperative laboratory screening tests necessary to evaluate ambulatory surgical patients? *Surgery* 1988;**104**:639–45.

30 Perez A, Planell J, Bacardaz C *et al.* Value of routine preoperative tests: a multicentre study in four general hospitals. *Br J Anaesth* 1995;**74**:250–6.

31 Golub R, Cantu R, Sorrento JJ, Stein HD. Efficacy of preadmission testing in ambulatory surgical patients. *Am J Surg* 1992;**163**:565–71.

32 Munro J, Booth A, Nicholl J. Routine preoperative testing: a systematic review of the evidence. *Health Technol Assess* 1997;**1**(12):1–62.

33 Fischer SP. Development and effectiveness of an anesthesia preoperative evaluation clinic in a teaching hospital. *Anesthesiology* 1996;**85**:196–206.

34 Carson JL, Poses RM, Spence RK, Bonavita G. Severity of anaemia and operative mortality and morbidity. *Lancet* 1988;**I**:727–9.

35 Rogers ZR, Powars DR, Kinney TR, Williams WD, Schroeder WA. Nonblack patients with sickle cell disease have African beta S gene cluster haplotypes. *JAMA* 1989;**261**:2991–4.

36 Wong E-M, Tillyer ML, Saunders PRI. Pre-operative screening for sickle cell trait in adult day surgery; is it necessary? *Amb Surg* 1996;**4**:41–5.

37 Campbell IT, Gosling P. Preoperative biochemical screening. Routine urine test is good enough in patients under 50 (editorial). *Br Med J* 1988;**297**:803–4.

38 Callaghan LC, Edwards ND, Reilly CS. Utilisation of the pre-operative ECG. *Anaesthesia* 1995;**50**:488–90.

39 Gold BS, Young ML, Kinman JL, Kitz DS, Berlin J, Schwartz JS. The utility of preoperative electrocardiograms in the ambulatory surgical patient. *Arch Intern Med* 1992;**152**:301–5.

40 Goldberger AL, O'Konski M. Utility of the routine electrocardiogram before surgery and on general hospital admission. Critical review and new guidelines. *Ann Int Med* 1986;**105**:552–7.

41 Pollard JB, Zboray AL, Mazze RI. Economic benefits attributed to opening a preoperative evaluation clinic for outpatients. *Anesth Analg* 1996;**83**:407–10.

42 Twersky RS, Lebovits AH, Lewis M, Frank D. Early anesthesia evaluation of the ambulatory surgical patient: does it really help? *J Clin Anesth* 1992;**4**:204–7.

43   Claxton AR, Lindsay SA, Watts JC, Smith I. Ambulatory anesthesia practices in the United Kingdom. *Sem Anesth* 1997;**16**:178–88.
44   Koay CB, Marks NJ. A nurse-led pre-admission clinic for elective ENT surgery–the first eight months. *Ann R Coll Surg Eng* 1996;**78**:15–19.
45   Royal College of Anaesthetists. *Guidelines for the provision of anaesthetic services.* London: Royal College of Anaesthetists, 1999.
46   American Society of Anesthesiologists Task Force on Preoperative Fasting. Practice guidelines for preoperative fasting and the use of pharmacologic agents to reduce the risk of pulmonary aspiration: application to healthy patients undergoing elective procedures. *Anesthesiology* 1999;**90**:896–905.
47   Phillips S, Hutchinson S, Davidson T. Preoperative drinking does not affect gastric contents. *Br J Anaesth* 1993;**70**:6–9.
48   Hargreaves J. Benzodiazepine premedication in minor day-case surgery: comparison of oral midazolam and temazepam with placebo. *Br J Anaesth* 1988;**61**:611–16.
49   Nightingale JJ, Norman J. A comparison of midazolam and temazepam for premedication of day case patients. *Anaesthesia* 1988;**43**:111–13.
50   Philip BK. Hazards of amnesia after midazolam in ambulatory surgical patients (letter). *Anesth Analg* 1987;**66**:97–8.
51   Raybould D, Bradshaw EG. Premedication for day case surgery. A study of oral midazolam. *Anaesthesia* 1987;**42**:591–5.
52   Obey PA, Ogg TW, Gilks WR. Temazepam and recovery in day surgery. *Anaesthesia* 1988;**43**:49–51.
53   Bailie R, Christmas L, Price N, Restall J, Simpson P, Wesnes K. Effects of temazepam premedication on cognitive recovery following alfentanil-propofol anaesthesia. *Br J Anaesth* 1989;**63**:68–75.
54   Sanders LD, Piggot SE, Isaac PA *et al.* Reversal of benzodiazepine sedation with the antagonist flumazenil. *Br J Anaesth* 1991;**66**:445–53.
55   Manchikanti L, Roush JR. Effect of preanesthetic glycopyrrolate and cimetidine on gastric fluid pH and volume in outpatients. *Anesth Analg* 1984;**63**:40–6.
56   Duffy BL. Regurgitation during pelvic laparoscopy. *Br J Anaesth* 1979;**51**:1089–90.
57   Lam AM, Grace DM, Manninen PH, Diamond C. The effects of cimetidine and ranitidine with and without metoclopramide on gastric volume and pH in morbidly obese patients. *Can Anaesth Soc J* 1986;**33**:773–9.
58   Boulay K, Blanloeil Y, Bourveau M, Geay G, Malinovsky J. Effects of oral ranitidine, famotidine and omeprazole on gastric volume and pH at induction and recovery from general anaesthesia. *Br J Anaesth* 1994;**73**:475–8.
59   Rosenblum M, Weller RS, Conard PL, Falvey EA, Gross JB. Ibuprofen provides longer lasting analgesia than fentanyl after laparoscopic surgery. *Anesth Analg* 1991;**73**:255–9.
60   Code WE, Yip RW, Rooney ME, Browne PM, Herz T. Preoperative naproxen sodium reduces postoperative pain following arthroscopic knee surgery. *Can J Anaesth* 1994;**41**:98–101.

2: Principles of general anaesthesia

ALEXANDER P L GOODWIN

Overview

Although many day surgery procedures may be performed under local or regional anaesthesia, with or without sedation, general anaesthesia remains extremely popular with patients, their anaesthetists, and surgeons. This chapter will review some of the key aspects which are required to deliver safe and efficient general anaesthesia.

Consideration will be given to the facilities in which general anaesthesia is provided to day case patients, including freestanding units. The relative advantages and disadvantages of a separate anaesthetic induction room will be discussed. Minimum monitoring standards and record keeping will be addressed.

Much of this chapter will deal with the conduct of general anaesthesia. Although the specific drugs and techniques for inhalation and intravenous anaesthesia will be considered later in separate chapters, this chapter will consider premedication, co-induction, neuromuscular blocking drugs, management of the airway, temperature control, and perioperative fluid management. The specific problems associated with laparoscopy will be addressed as well as the more general hazards associated with various patient positions. The chapter will conclude with a consideration of infection control, sterilisation, and disinfection.

Introduction

In the middle of the 19th century the first general anaesthetics were for day case dental extractions. One hundred and fifty years later, general anaesthesia remains the mainstay of day case anaesthesia. The quality of general anaesthesia is possibly the most important part of the patient's day surgery episode. Without quality, morbidity increases and patient satisfaction decreases. The outcomes by which general anaesthesia for day surgery might be judged are difficult to define. Rapid trouble-free immediate recovery may not equate with a good outcome once the patient is discharged. Possible outcome measures are listed in Box 2.1.

Box 2.1 Outcome measures of day surgery anaesthesia

- Immediate recovery–time to eye opening
- First-stage recovery–time in recovery room
- Incidence of postoperative nausea and vomiting
- Other postoperative morbidity
- Time to discharge home
- Unplanned admission to an inpatient bed
- Ability to carry out more complex surgery on day case basis
- Patient satisfaction
- Return to normal activity
- Cost effectiveness

Day surgery general anaesthesia is not merely the administration of drugs that produce the anaesthetic triad of hypnosis, analgesia, and lack of reflex activity; it is a process involving the organisation of resources to ensure the safety of the patient and the highest quality of care. This chapter sets out to discuss the process of general anaesthesia.

Preparation and organisation

Preparation for day surgery general anaesthesia begins in the general practitioner's surgery with appropriate selection. It continues into the outpatient clinic where further screening and the provision of adequate information will contribute to the patient's overall experience. Preoperative assessment and visit to the day surgery unit prior to the day of admission is another tool in the reduction in patient preoperative anxiety and an aid in increasing patient satisfaction.

Facilities

In the United Kingdom most day surgery units occupy dedicated facilities within the environs of a hospital. The units are used solely for the delivery of care on a day stay basis. Although North America has seen the proliferation of freestanding day surgery centres away from the hospital campus, this has yet to occur to a significant degree in the UK. The pattern in the remainder of Europe is variable. The British Association of Day Surgery (BADS) has made recommendations for free-standing units; these are outlined in Box 2.2.

Box 2.2 The British Association for Day Surgery recommendations for freestanding units

- A medical member of staff should remain on the premises until all day cases are discharged.
- The nursing staff and operating department assistants should be experienced in day surgery. They should be trained in operating theatre technique, anaesthesia, and recovery.
- A preoperative assessment facility should be provided.
- An arrangement with an inpatient hospital should be established in the event of emergency admissions.
- Transport arrangements for emergency transfers to an inpatient hospital should be established.
- A quality assurance programme should be in place.

Design

Day surgery theatre design should conform to all statutory requirements for operating theatres. Full recovery facilities must be adjacent to the operating room.

Anaesthetic rooms

Opinions on the value of an anaesthetic room remain polarised on a geographical basis. Whilst common in Europe, the anaesthetic room is rare in North America. Anaesthetic rooms were originally built to spare patients the sight of things that might otherwise shock and distress them.[1] This concept was universally accepted and operating theatres worldwide were designed to include anaesthetic rooms. In America in the 1970s the use of anaesthetic rooms declined and they have subsequently disappeared from building programmes. Day surgery patients are well prepared and the argument that unpleasant sights would shock them may be invalid. The suggested advantages and disadvantages of the anaesthetic room are listed in Box 2.3.

Box 2.3 The relative advantages and disadvantages of anaesthetic induction rooms

Advantages	*Disadvantages*
• Pleasant, calm room	• Increased risk to patient
• Increased patient turnover	• Greater capital cost
• Trainee supervision	• Duplication of equipment
• Local anaesthetic techniques	• Mandatory disconnection of patient
• Prevents delay in theatre cleaning, etc.	• Complicated record keeping
• Better for accompanying parents	• Patients cannot position themselves
• Adequate work surfaces	• Less help available
• Proximity of drugs and equipment	

In times of financial stringency few hospitals can provide minimal monitoring standards in both anaesthetic rooms and the operating theatres. However, many anaesthetists commence anaesthesia in the operating theatre in patients considered to be "at risk", such as those with major systemic diseases or women undergoing caesarean section. One therefore questions whether all patients should have anaesthesia induced, fully and continuously monitored, in the operating theatre, particularly as induction is one of the most hazardous times during a patient's anaesthetic. It is the author's practice to allow patients to walk into the operating theatre and position themselves on the operating table. The key to success is the change in culture that makes this practice the norm for all the day surgery team. Day surgery lends itself to this cultural change. Subsequently, it has been shown that anxiety levels differ little relating to where anaesthesia is induced.[2]

Parental involvement in the induction of anaesthesia can be of particular benefit in preschool children (Chapter 9). However, parents should not be forced to be present as this has been shown to increase parental anxiety.[3] Anxious parents increase anxiety in their children.

Monitoring and record keeping

Patient monitoring should be to the same standard as that employed for inpatient surgery. The Association of Anaesthetists of Great Britain and Ireland has described what it considers to be minimal monitoring standards (Box 2.4).[4] Other national bodies have produced similar guidelines. The anaesthetist should always be present throughout the conduct of the whole anaesthetic and should ensure that an adequate record of the procedure is made. Monitoring should be commenced before induction of anaesthesia and continued until the patient has recovered from the anaesthetic. The anaesthetic machine must be monitored. The frequency of measurement of patient variables should be appropriate to the clinical state of the patient. In healthy day surgery patients this frequency will probably be every five minutes whilst the patient is physiologically stable. A peripheral nerve stimulator should be readily available when neuromuscular blocking drugs are employed. Additional monitoring may be required as the length of operations increases or for patients with co-existing disease. Adequate monitoring should always be applied, even during anaesthesia of brief duration or when using local anaesthetics or sedation techniques which may lead to loss of consciousness or to cardiovascular or respiratory suppression. Anaesthetists should issue clear instructions concerning monitoring of postoperative care when handing the patient over to recovery ward staff.

Monitoring depth of anaesthesia
Intraoperative awareness occurs relatively rarely but is much feared by patients. Clinical signs do not always reliably reflect anaesthetic "depth"

Box 2.4 Minimal monitoring standards recommended by the Association of Anaesthetists of Great Britain and Ireland

(1) Anaesthetist's presence throughout
(2) Monitoring of anaesthetic machine:
   - Oxygen supply
   - Breathing system
(3) Monitoring the patient
   - Clinical observations:
       Patient's colour
       Response to surgical stimulus
       Chest wall movement
       Palpation of pulse
       Auscultation of heart and breath sounds
   - Continuous monitoring devices:
       Pulse volume
       Arterial blood pressure
       Arterial oxygen saturation
       Electrocardiogram
       Expired volume, carbon dioxide, and airway pressure
       Monitoring of body temperature where appropriate
Monitoring should be continuous throughout the period of induction, anaesthesia, and recovery

and a more specific monitor has long been sought. Awareness should be reflected by changes in brain electrical activity but any subtle differences are swamped by the mass of data within the raw EEG. Various processed parameters have been investigated but these have usually shown anaesthetic-specific effects and a poor degree of reproducibility. Auditory evoked potentials are undergoing extensive clinical trials, with promising early results,[5] although a commercial monitor is still some way off.

One potential anaesthetic depth monitor which is commercially available is the Bispectral Index (BIS), which processes the EEG to produce a numerical value ranging from 0 to 100. Validation of the BIS has been difficult but it appears able to discriminate between the awake and unconscious states. There is reasonable evidence that most patients will be reliably unaware if the BIS is 60 or below,[6, 7] although there is probably some individual variability. Nevertheless, several investigators have attempted to use BIS to refine their anaesthetic titration so that patients remain unaware but receive less anaesthesia, thereby reducing costs and improving recovery times. For example, titrating propofol to a BIS value of 45–60 (increased to 60–75 towards the end of anaesthesia) reduced propofol requirements and hastened early recovery compared to conventional drug delivery.[8] Similarly, titrating inhaled anaesthesia to a BIS of 60 reduced anaesthetic consumption by 31–38% and shortened awakening times by 20–50% compared to normal clinical practice, which resulted in average BIS values of 42.[9] Of some concern was the finding that the BIS-titrated groups required more neuromuscular blocking drugs during the procedure.[9] This may have reflected increased movement, suggesting inadequate anaesthesia, although there may simply have been less potentiation of neuromuscular block from the reduced volatile anaesthetic dose. Other workers have shown that BIS does not reliably predict intraoperative patient movement (a clinical sign usually taken to indicate inadequate anaesthesia) and that BIS values at the end of anaesthesia do not correlate with rates of awakening.[10] Until the reliability of the BIS is better understood, using it to reduce anaesthetic consumption will almost certainly reduce the margin of safety by which awareness is prevented. The best safeguard against intraoperative awareness remains the avoidance of neuromuscular blocking drugs (see below).

Record keeping

Record keeping, whilst not an absolute legal requirement, makes professional survival in the ever-increasing litigious society much easier. There is no standard anaesthetic record in the United Kingdom. In recent years, however, both the Royal College of Anaesthetists and the Association of Anaesthetists of Great Britain and Ireland have set out what they regard as the minimum data set for an anaesthetic record. The General Medical Council has also laid down, for assessment purposes, what it considers to be essential recorded information. While the format of the anaesthetic record is a matter for local preference, the suggested contents are shown in Box 2.5.

Automatic record keeping might help in the day surgery setting where turnover of cases is rapid. At present, automated record-keeping systems are uncommon in British day surgery units. Computerised records would provide detailed information about both individual and departmental practice. These are most valuable for auditing specific areas of anaesthetic care. However, the patient's notes remain confidential documents and disclosure of information for research, teaching, and audit may raise ethical problems unless consent is obtained or the data have been effectively anonymised. A major problem with automated record-keeping systems is how to integrate information on drug dosage, interventions, technique, and events with the automatically recorded parameters. At present, this usually requires a considerable amount of information to be entered using a keyboard, which is time consuming and distracting in the day care setting.

Conduct of anaesthesia

Premedication

Sedative premedicants are rarely given prior to day case anaesthesia. However, there is no doubt that for specific situations the use of a "premed"

Box 2.5 Recommended minimal data set for the anaesthetic record. Based on the Royal College of Anaesthetists and the Association of Anaesthetists of Great Britain and Ireland's good practice guidelines[40]

(1) **Basic data entry:** names of surgeon and anaesthetist, date, proposed operation
(2) **Patient identification:** name, age, gender, hospital number
(3) **Preoperative assessment:** relevant history, physical examination, drugs, allergies
(4) **Anaesthetic technique:** induction and maintenance technique used, including anaesthetic agents used recorded in detail
(5) **Intravenous drugs administered:** clear record of preoperative and intraoperative drugs given, doses, and times of administration
(6) **Equipment monitoring:** relevant equipment monitoring such as F_iO_2 (always) and pressure alarms
(7) **Patient monitoring used:** this should be in accordance with the recommendations of the Association of Anaesthetists or similar national body
(8) **Physiological variables recorded:** time-based chart recordings of relevant parameters including preinduction values
(9) **Frequency of recording of physiological variables:** frequent recording from induction depending on patient stability, but not less frequently than every 15 minutes for pulse, blood pressure, and oxygen saturation
(10) **Fluid balance:** evidence of venous cannulation and records of fluids administered and blood loss
(11) **Postoperative pain relief:** clear and appropriate postoperative analgesic orders
(12) **Other postoperative instructions:** oxygen therapy, immediate postoperative fluids, and monitoring to Association (or similar) standards
(13) **Critical incidents and complications should be accurately documented**
(14) **If a case is handed over to another anaesthetist this should be documented**
(15) **Unexpected admission to ICU or HDU:** the reasons for admission should be clearly documented

F_iO_2 inspired oxygen fraction; ICU, intensive care unit; HDU, high-dependency unit

may enhance the quality of the general anaesthesia without prolonging recovery.[11] Hypnosis has also been employed to reduce preoperative anxiety,[12] and even the preoperative anaesthetic visit may be helpful.

Premedication may also encompass other medications administered in the preoperative period. Prophylactic analgesia should be administered for any procedure expected to produce significant postoperative pain (see Chapter 7). Prophylactic antiemetics may also sometimes be given preoperatively. Most patients will not benefit from antacid or gastropropulsive medications, although these may be indicated in "high-risk" individuals.

Painless venous cannulation for children and phobic adults is possible with the use of local anaesthetic creams, provided that these are applied sufficiently early. Finally, regular medications for chronic diseases should generally also be administered prior to surgery (see Chapter 1).

Induction

A rapid recovery is important after day surgery. Induction agents should have a rapid onset of action and provide for a rapid recovery, cause no pain on injection, avoid histamine release and anaphylaxis and not induce involuntary movements. Induction of anaesthesia may be achieved with a variety of inhaled or intravenous (IV) anaesthetics (see Chapters 3 and 4). None of these is perfect in every respect.

The ideal IV agent should reliably and pleasantly induce anaesthesia within one arm-brain circulation. It should be free of side effects and wear off in a few minutes. It must be remembered that the injection of an IV anaesthetic drug into the circulation cannot be easily withdrawn, whereas inhalational agents may be more readily eliminated. Control of the airway is the most important factor when administering IV anaesthesia. The inability to safely manage an airway is an absolute contraindication to the use of IV anaesthesia.

An audit from Cambridge in the mid-1990s suggested that propofol was used in 95% of day cases and the remaining 5% were induced using an inhalational method.[42] Propofol remains extremely popular, although the proportion of inhalation inductions may now have increased slightly.

Co-induction
Co-induction involves the use of adjunctive medications to reduce the dose of the anaesthetic induction agent. This practice may also improve haemodynamic stability. The most commonly used co-induction agent is midazolam, in a dose of 0.03–0.06 mg/kg (2–4 mg for an average adult). Administering midazolam approximately two minutes prior to induction may reduce the dose of propofol required by as much as half, especially if an opioid such as alfentanil is given with midazolam. It was initially thought that a co-induction dose of midazolam did not significantly delay recovery. More recent evidence suggests that midazolam impairs postoperative psychomotor performance[13] and discharge may even be delayed.[14]

Because of this concern, the concept of auto co-induction has been introduced. This involves administering propofol 0.4 mg/kg (typically 20–30 mg) two minutes before the main induction dose. Although the anaesthetic-sparing effect is not as great as that of midazolam, auto co-induction still reduces propofol requirements by more than 20% and decreases the degree of hypotension and apnoea.[14] In contrast to midazolam co-induction, recovery times are unaffected by this technique.

40

Maintenance

Total intravenous anaesthesia (TIVA) became practicable in the early 1970s with the advent of non-barbiturate induction agents and has become more common with the introduction of propofol (see Chapter 4). TIVA may be used for general anaesthesia, as well as for sedation during regional block (see Chapter 6). Intravenous anaesthetics are often also used as the major hypnotic component in combination with gaseous agents, especially nitrous oxide. Inhalation anaesthesia is still commonly used during day surgery (see Chapter 3), especially since the availability of less soluble anaesthetics and a resumption of interest in inhalation induction.

Box 2.6 Specific checks when undertaking intravenous or inhaled anaesthesia

Intravenous anaesthesia	• Correctly functioning infusion pump(s) • Battery back-up in case of mains supply failure • Empty syringe warning • Occlusion warning • Dedicated intravenous cannula with Luer lock connections to prevent disconnection • Intravenous cannula in clear view for monitoring • Caution with mixtures of intravenous drugs which may interact • A proper syringe refill system
Inhalation anaesthesia	• Agent-specific calibrated vaporiser • Full vaporiser, sight glass in clear view • Leak test anaesthesia machine after siting vaporiser • Check vaporiser filler cap is correctly seated • Correctly functioning scavenging system • End-expired agent monitoring (to confirm drug delivery)

Whatever method of general anaesthesia is used, a variety of precautions should be taken. These include a thorough check of the anaesthesia machine before use, full resuscitation equipment, and normal minimal monitoring. Additional checks will be required for either IV or inhaled anaesthesia, as shown in Box 2.6. Great care must be taken to ensure that sufficient anaesthetic is actually being delivered. This is facilitated by end-expired agent monitoring with inhalation anaesthesia, but will require careful observation of the infusion pump, syringe, and cannula with IV anaesthesia. The target controlled infusion system (see Chapter 4) using propofol has addressed some of the potential problems of IV anaesthesia.

Nevertheless, awareness may be a problem if inadequate anaesthesia is supplied in the presence of neuromuscular block. Factors contributing to awareness are listed in Box 2.7.

Box 2.7 Factors contributing to awareness under general anaesthesia. Not all are relevant to the day care setting

Equipment	• Lack of monitoring • Failure of drug delivery systems • Leaks in anaesthesia machine/breathing system • Ventilator failure
Technique	• Forget to turn on delivery system • Lack of analgesia • Lack of premedication • Reliance on opioids • Reliance on nitrous oxide • Reliance on neuromuscular blocking drugs • Miscalculation of anaesthetic dose • Delay, due to difficult intubation, etc.
Patient	• Natural variation in sensitivity to anaesthetic agent • Past history of awareness • Drug addicts • Alcoholics • Young patients • Very sick and emergency cases
Operation	• Bronchoscopy • Cardiopulmonary bypass • Caesarean section

Nitrous oxide

Nitrous oxide (N_2O) is a weak anaesthetic agent but a potent analgesic. It is cheap, reduces the risk of awareness and reduces the requirements for, and hence the cost of, other anaesthetic agents. The use of N_2O remains controversial, however, especially because of its effect on postoperative nausea and vomiting (PONV). Two metaanalyses[15, 16] concluded that N_2O increased emesis in susceptible patients and operations associated with an increased incidence of PONV. Three mechanisms have been postulated as contributing to an increase in PONV with N_2O.

(1)   Increased gastrointestinal distension.
(2)   Changes in middle ear pressure and stimulation of the vestibular apparatus.
(3)   Stimulation of the sympathetic nervous system.

Despite these effects, a number of studies in patients at lower baseline risk for PONV have failed to show any significant benefit from omitting N_2O.[17, 18]

Neuromuscular blocking drugs

It is the author's view that neuromuscular blocking drugs have a limited role in day case anaesthesia. The introduction of the laryngeal mask airway (LMA) has reduced dramatically the situations where neuromuscular blocking drugs are required. Neuromuscular blocking drugs are only indicated for the establishment of a safe and protected airway, as for example in patients who may require a rapid-sequence induction in the presence of a symptomatic hiatus hernia and in situations where significant muscle relaxation is necessary for surgical access (e.g. laparoscopic cholecystectomy). Some authors have advocated the use of propofol and alfentanil for intubation. Excellent intubating conditions were produced in 86% of patients providing enough propofol was given to produce jaw relaxation.[19] Inhalation induction with sevoflurane can also provide satisfactory tracheal intubating conditions.[20]

The ideal neuromuscular blocking drug for day case surgery provides rapid onset and offset of effect. No single neuromuscular blocking drug available today provides these properties without detrimental side effects. Succinylcholine (suxamethonium) has the shortest onset and offset time but its significant side effect of muscle pains is a major concern to day surgery patients. Severe postoperative myalgia may delay a patient's recovery and prevent them from returning to work in the immediate postoperative period.

Atracurium and vecuronium are intermediate-acting neuromuscular blocking drugs that have similar pharmacodynamic properties; their onset time is 2–4 minutes and their recovery index (time from 25% to 75% recovery of neuromuscular function) is >10 minutes. Cisatracurium is similar in action to atracurium but with a slower onset time and less histamine release.[21] To minimise an unnecessary long duration in day surgery, initial doses may be reduced, although this will further delay the onset of action.

Newer neuromuscular blocking drugs include rocuronium which has a rapid onset of action and a similar duration of action to vecuronium. Mivacurium is a short-acting agent which has been used in day surgery. Its recovery index is only four minutes. This means that spontaneous recovery of neuromuscular function is as quick as neostigmine-induced recovery following the use of atracurium and vecuronium. The onset time is similar to atracurium and vecuronium but histamine release is common. In the near future, rapacuronium should be available. This is a non-depolarising neuromuscular blocking drug which combines a rapid onset with a brief duration of action. Although not quite a "non-depolarising version of succinylcholine", rapacuronium may combine the duration of mivacurium with the onset time of rocuronium.[22]

Reversal of neuromuscular block

Failure to reverse neuromuscular block, even with mivacurium, may result in residual weakness. However, it has been suggested that glycopyrrolate and neostigmine increase PONV,[23] especially when high doses are used.[24] Glycopyrrolate does not cross the blood–brain barrier to the same extent as atropine. The use of glycopyrrolate may reduce the incidence of central cholinergic effects such as delayed recovery and short-term memory loss.[18,25] The reduction in the use of non-depolarising neuromuscular blocking drugs in day surgery has reduced the need for pharmacological reversal and its possible side effects. Smaller doses of neuromuscular blocking drugs, together with the use of propofol and short-acting opioids, may also reduce the need for reversal in those cases that might require muscle relaxation. Adequate relaxation of muscles for most day surgery procedures may be achieved using inhaled anaesthetics.

Airway management

Three common methods of airway management are available to the day surgery anaesthetist: the facemask, the LMA, and the endotracheal tube. Whilst the endotracheal tube remains the gold standard in airway management, the LMA has brought many advantages over both the facemask and endotracheal tube to everyday anaesthetic practice.

The LMA was designed in 1981 by Dr A I J Brain as part of a search for an airway that was more practical than a facemask but less invasive than an endotracheal tube. The first prototype was the marriage of a Goldman dental mask and a size 10 endotracheal tube. The design objective was to provide an end-to-end airtight seal around the larynx without violating sphincters, thus offering a more physiological approach to airway control than endotracheal intubation. The LMA is made of medical-grade silicone rubber and is entirely latex free.

Since the launch of the LMA in 1988 there have been more than 1800 publications on the use and misuse of the device. Brain has emphasised that proper patient selection and correct insertion technique can best avoid problems. Several large epidemiological surveys have confirmed the safety and efficacy of the LMA for both spontaneous and controlled ventilation in properly selected fasted patients.[26, 27]

Originally the LMA was thought to be a "hands-free" replacement for the facemask. It is now used in many patients that would traditionally have been managed with an endotracheal tube. Advantages of the LMA over the facemask and endotracheal tube are listed in Box 2.8.

Box 2.8 Advantages and disadvantages of the LMA over the facemask and endotracheal tube which have been demonstrated by prospective, randomised controlled trials modified from reference[41]. With permission.

Laryngeal mask compared to tracheal tube

Advantages

- Placement quicker for anaesthetists
- Less haemodynamic stimulation during insertion and removal
- Intraocular pressure rise less during insertion
- Frequency of cough is less during emergence
- Oxygen saturation higher during emergence
- Incidence of postoperative sore throat is less in adults
- Airways better tolerated
- Voice less affected

Disadvantages

- Gastric insufflation more likely
- Air leak more likely

Laryngeal mask compared to facemask

Advantages

- Oxygen saturations higher
- Surgical conditions superior for minor ENT surgery in children
- Hand fatigue less

Disadvantages

- Frequency of oesophageal reflux higher

The LMA also comes in a flexible, reinforced form, used commonly in head and neck surgery. A version of the LMA to assist in managing the difficult airway is also now available (LMA-Fastrach™), although this is likely to have only a limited place in day surgery. A prototype LMA that isolates the gastrointestinal and respiratory tract and offers a higher seal pressure is undergoing clinical trials. Other developments include the provision of single and multiple reflectance pulse oximeter probes on the LMA cuff. This would provide a measure of central oxygen saturation and tissue perfusion.

The cuffed oropharyngeal airway (COPA)

Extratracheal airways have become increasingly popular for spontaneously breathing patients undergoing minor and intermediate day case surgery. The COPA is a modified Guedel airway with an inflatable distal cuff and a proximal 15 mm connector for attachment to the anaesthetic breathing system. Clinical experience with this device remains limited. Most published studies show few, if any, advantages over the LMA and in many cases the airway achieved with the COPA is significantly inferior.

Laparoscopy

Although the physiological effects of laparoscopy may compromise patients with moderate to severe co-existing disease, in the day surgery setting, the physiological changes are reversible and few adverse clinical events occur. Traditionally, airway management during gynaecological laparoscopy has been with the endotracheal tube. Intermittent positive pressure ventilation and a cuffed endotracheal tube are used to protect the patient against the physiological changes during laparoscopy and the potential intraoperative risks. The Trendelenburg position and the increased abdominal pressure from peritoneal insufflation with carbon dioxide in laparoscopy can cause cardiovascular and respiratory changes as listed in Box 2.9.

Box 2.9 Physiological changes during laparoscopy

- Reduced total lung compliance
- Reduced functional residual capacity
- Altered ventilation/perfusion ratio
- Splanchnic and aortocaval compression, reduced venous return
- Increased systemic vascular resistance
- Reduced cardiac output
- Vagal stimulation
- Hypercarbia, potential for acidosis

As a consequence of the physiological changes and surgical insult, a variety of intraoperative risks may be encountered (Box 2.10).

Box 2.10 Intraoperative risks of laparoscopy

Anaesthetic	• Hypotension
	• Hypertension
	• Dysrhythmias
	• Hypoventilation
	• Reflux of stomach contents
	• Pulmonary aspiration
	• Neuropathy as a result of positioning
Surgical	• Perforation of blood vessels
	• Perforation of bowel
	• Gas embolism
	• Pneumothorax
	• Pneumomediastinum
	• Pneumopericardium
	• Laparotomy

The main issues affecting anaesthetists are the risks of aspiration, hypoventilation, dysrhythmias, and peripheral neuropathies. The mechanism for an increase in reflux and aspiration in a healthy patient is not based on sound scientific evidence. The Trendelenburg position does not reduce lower oesophageal sphincter tone[28] and the use of neuromuscular block does not reduce intraabdominal pressure.[29]

A postal survey of 243 UK hospitals revealed that approximately 60% of experienced anaesthetists used the LMA for gynaecological laparoscopy.[30] The results of large-scale epidemiological studies[26] support the findings of controlled trials[31, 32] that the LMA is a safe method of airway management in gynaecological laparoscopy. However, the safety of this technique depends on a short operating time, close intraoperative monitoring, and the presence of an experienced anaesthetist and surgeon. A "rule of 15s" has been suggested for LMA usage in anaesthesia for laparoscopy: less than 15° of table tilt, less than 15 minutes operative time, and an intraabdominal pressure of less than 15 cmH$_2$O.

Intravenous fluids

The routine use of fluids in day surgery anaesthesia is controversial. A much-quoted study[33] showed a reduction in drowsiness, dizziness, headache, and thirst, together with a subjective feeling of well-being following the administration of 2 litres of fluid perioperatively. However, these patients were anaesthetised with thiopental (thiopentone) and halothane, anaesthetics which are no longer commonly used. With propofol alone or with newer inhaled anaesthetics, the benefit of fluids in procedures lasting less than 20 minutes is uncertain. However, less thirst, drowsiness, dizziness, and nausea have been reported in patients receiving 20 ml/kg of isotonic solution during gynaecological surgery lasting 30 minutes.[34] Reduction in thirst by either reducing the preoperative fast or administering intraoperative fluids may reduce the incidence of postoperative vomiting.

Temperature maintenance

As day surgery procedures become more complex and the acceptable operating time increases, it is important to maintain patients' body temperature. Perioperative hypothermia is common in surgical patients.[35] The principal cause is core-to-peripheral redistribution of body heat as a result of impairment of central thermoregulation by anaesthesia. Cool ambient temperatures and the administration of room temperature fluids accelerate heat loss to the environment. Randomised controlled trials have shown that mild hypothermia increases the incidence of wound infection and prolongs hospitalisation, increases the incidence of morbid cardiac events and ventricular tachycardia and impairs coagulation. Other complications include enhanced anaesthetic drug effects, prolonged recovery room stays, shivering and impaired immune function.[36]

The most effective means of preventing perioperative hypothermia is active warming. High ambient temperatures, warmed intravenous fluids, and active cutaneous warming are useful intraoperatively. Warm air blowers such as the Bair Hugger™ are extremely efficient in maintaining body temperature. Temperature should be monitored during prolonged cases. Active cutaneous warming and intravenous pethidine (meperidine) both abolish postoperative shivering, which is distressing to patients and can adversely affect outcome. Thermal management may reduce complications and improve outcome in more complex day surgical patients. The cost effectiveness of perioperative warming has yet to be established, however.

Recovery

Emergence from anaesthesia is potentially hazardous and patients require close observation until recovery is complete. In order to facilitate the smooth running of an operating list, the anaesthetist transfers accountability for the patient's immediate care to staff who have been trained in recovery procedures. Close collaboration between surgeon and anaesthetist is required at this time, in order that clear instructions are given to the recovery staff.

Following general anaesthesia, the patient is normally placed in the recovery position on a tipping trolley or bed and escorted to the recovery area by the anaesthetist. A full summary of the patient's treatment and all paperwork should be handed to the recovery staff. The anaesthetist should ensure that the recovery staff are happy to take responsibility for the patient before care is transferred.

All staff who work in recovery rooms must be educated and trained to the highest professional standards. They can then provide optimum care for patients and respond to the potentially life-threatening circumstances that may arise at any moment. The range and complexity of modern anaesthesia and surgery have extended the possibilities for successful treatment but, paradoxically, have also increased the hazards and thus the responsibilities of recovery staff.

Each hospital should develop standards for patient care and draw up written guidelines for as many aspects of the specialised work of the recovery room as is deemed necessary. Standards should be audited regularly and guidelines reviewed and revised as appropriate. Recovery staff should maintain close links with other staff involved in patient care. Recommendations for recovery room equipment and further discussion of the recovery process may be found in Chapter 8.

Operating room practice

Operating room practice in the day surgery setting is essentially the same as that in inpatient operating theatres. The principal differences are the patient and the geography of the pre- and postoperative areas which, in a self-contained unit, are in the same location. This provides benefits to patients and staff.

Patient movement and positioning[37]

Care is of paramount importance when moving and positioning both the anaesthetised and awake patient. An anaesthetised patient has reduced sympathetic reflexes and hence may react adversely to minor changes in body posture. This is particularly true of hypovolaemic patients and those undergoing regional anaesthesia. All movements should be smooth and gentle.

A variety of positions may expose patients to risk.

Trendelenburg position (head-down tilt)

- In the obese patient there may be a reduction in lung volumes.
- Cyanosis may occur in plethoric patients, even with adequate ventilation.
- If the arm has to be abducted, this should be no greater than 90°, with the elbow slightly flexed and the forearm pronated to prevent traction on the brachial plexus. The head should be turned towards the side of the abducted arm. The abducted arm should not be allowed to fall below the level of the body.
- An increase in cerebral venous pressure will reduce cerebral perfusion pressure; care should be taken to maintain blood pressure.
- Prolonged Trendelenburg position can cause cerebral oedema and retinal detachment.

Prone position

- Functional residual capacity is increased.
- The pelvis and shoulders should be supported so that breathing is not unduly interfered with and that all pressure is removed from the abdomen and the inferior *vena cava*. Many use a cuffed endotracheal tube although some experienced anaesthetists use an armoured LMA.
- Skeletal damage easily occurs in the unconscious patient, particularly when being turned.
- Care should be taken when moving arms, as shoulders may be dislocated.
- Eyes should be protected to avoid corneal abrasions and blindness. Retinal artery occlusion has been reported.

Lithotomy and Lloyd-Davies

- Move both legs together to avoid strain on pelvic ligaments.
- If legs are on the inside of poles, pressure may be exerted on the lateral popliteal nerves.
- Hip flexion may stretch the sciatic nerve.
- Bilateral compartment syndrome has occurred after several hours in the lithotomy position.

Lateral position

- Ventilation perfusion mismatch, especially with controlled ventilation.
- Nerve damage if careless.

Supine position

- Pressure on, and stretching of, nerves of arm, particularly the ulnar nerve.
- *Tendo Achilles* must not rest on the edge of the table.
- A soft pad raising the heels off the bed may lessen the incidence of venous thrombosis.
- A lumbar support may reduce the incidence of backache following surgery.

Infection control

Infection control is in the interests of both patients and staff. There is an absolute need to prevent the spread of pathogenic agents. The key areas of infection control are listed in Box 2.11.

Box 2.11 Key areas of infection control

- Ventilation of operating theatre
- Control of temperature and humidity
- Regular cleaning and sterilisation
- Appropriate clothing
- Regular hand washing
- Appropriate behaviour

Ventilation
The number of microorganisms in the air of an operating room depends on the size of the room, the amount of activity, the number of persons, and the rate at which the air is replaced. Current recommendations require 20–25 air changes per hour, with five of these being clean air. This ensures the removal of pollutants. Airflow is maintained by positive pressure and this system relies on all the doors being closed.[38]

Temperature and humidity
The recommended range of temperature in the operating room is 20–24°C.
Humidity should be 50–55%. It will be necessary to raise the temperature
above 24°C for paediatric cases. As temperature increases, so does the
growth of microorganisms. As well as maintaining a comfortable working
environment, the maintenance of recommended temperatures reduces the
growth of microorganisms.

Cleaning
Damp dusting at the start of the day removes dust particles and therefore
reduces bacteria levels. Newer operating rooms with modern ventilation
systems may not require damp dusting as the ventilation system will be efficient enough to keep bacterial levels down. All furniture and equipment
that has been in contact with a patient is considered contaminated and must
be cleaned prior to its next use.

Remember disinfectants kill microorganisms and are used on inanimate
objects. Antiseptics kill or inhibit growth of microorganisms and are sufficiently non-toxic to be applied to living tissues. Following an infected case,
the equipment is cleaned as usual and then the recommended disinfectant
(as per hospital policy) is applied and left to dry.

Sterilisation
Sterilisation is the complete killing of all microorganisms. All microorganisms, including spores, must be destroyed during the sterilisation
process. The method of sterilisation (Box 2.12) depends on the product or
article to be sterilised. The majority of operating instruments may be sterilised in an autoclave following decontamination. An autoclave uses steam
under pressure, allowing temperatures that kill organisms to be reached.
Delicate items such as catheters can be sterilised using γ radiation. This
method is expensive and usually associated with single-use, commercially
prepared items. The use of ethylene dioxide is also expensive and requires a
long sterilisation cycle (2–5 hours) as well as a long time for aeration. This
method may be used for items that cannot withstand the high temperature
and pressure of the autoclave.

Box 2.12 Methods of sterilisation

(1) Wet heat sterilisation: 121°C for 15 minutes, 134°C for 3 minutes
(2) Low-temperature steam and formaldehyde: 72–80°C for 1–2 hours
(3) Chemical sterilisation with ethylene oxide: 50°C for 1–16 hours
(4) Irradiation: 2.5 Mrad required to ensure sterility (γ rays)

Hand washing

The purpose of hand washing is to remove debris and transient microorganisms from the fingernails, hands, and forearms. This should reduce the resident microbial count to a minimum and inhibit rapid rebound growth of microorganisms. The most common scrub agents are chlorhexidine and betadine. Betadine (povidone iodine) is fast acting with a long duration of action. Iodine is present in very small concentrations, hence reducing the incidence of sensitisation. The length of the scrub procedure should be 3–5 minutes.

Clothing

All clothing used in the operating theatre should be designed and manufactured to limit, as much as possible, the airborne spread of bacteria and other microorganisms. At the same time, clothing needs to be comfortable and easy to launder. Tunics and trousers are generally worn. If dresses are worn, legs must be covered to prevent the shedding of skin scales. Fabrics used in the manufacture of operating theatre clothing should be lint free (to reduce dust and hence bacteria levels) and flame resistant. Cotton is not a suitable fabric as it sheds fibres and has an open weave, absorbing fluids. The use of facemasks to prevent airborne spread of infection has been questioned. Gould suggests that the use of masks makes no difference to infection rates.[39] Contamination of the wound, by droplets, may occur from members of the scrub team and therefore it is recommend that they should continue to wear masks. These recommendations apply only to those operating theatres with an efficient ventilation system.

Behaviour

Behaviour of operating theatre staff may affect infection rates. Movement around the operating theatre, respecting clean and dirty areas, keeping doors closed, and actually minimising movement all help to reduce the bacterial count. Correct use of operating theatre clothing and good aseptic technique are required. Universal precautions should be practised for all invasive procedures. This is to protect both patients and staff from exposure to bloodborne pathogens.

Quality assurance–standards and monitoring

Any day surgery unit should ensure that standards are set in accordance with recognised national guidelines and that these standards are monitored. Standards should be reflected in the mission statement and philosophy of the unit and should be a part of the objectives of the department. Staff should ensure that national and local patient standards are met where appropriate. The standards of Royal Colleges and other professional bodies should be adhered to. A local day surgery charter should be developed, particularly to include cancellations and a complaints procedure. Outlines of training, standards of care, and patient advice should be displayed.

The principal mode of monitoring standards will be by audit. Relevant national standards should be audited as part of a regular quality programme. Patient satisfaction survey results should be published and actioned. Quality assurance items should be regularly discussed. Audit and quality assurance items should be included in an annual report. Further information on quality of patient care and follow-up will be found in Chapter 8.

Summary

General anaesthesia remains a popular technique for day case surgery. It is important to ensure that the quality of general anaesthesia always reaches a high standard. Improvements in drugs, techniques, monitoring, and education have all increased the safety of general anaesthesia. Day surgery still requires the usual high standard of facilities with adequate monitoring and complete record keeping, irrespective of whether these are provided in a large hospital or a freestanding unit. Ensuring safe and continuous monitoring may require giving up the anaesthetic induction room, although this may be better tolerated by our patients than we might expect.

The vast majority of day case procedures may be achieved with spontaneous ventilation and the laryngeal mask. Even gynaecological laparoscopy may commonly be managed in this way. Tracheal intubation and the use of neuromuscular blocking drugs are not contraindicated, however, and may be required in certain circumstances. There are currently many neuromuscular blocking drugs to choose from, although none is ideal for day surgery. Use of the lowest dose necessary and trying to allow spontaneous recovery should minimise their associated problems.

As day surgery expands and more complex procedures are undertaken, many of the hazards previously faced by inpatients become increasingly important in the day care setting. Heat loss and redistribution may lead to hypothermia unless preventive measures are taken. Intraoperative dehydration may become problematic, although reduction in preoperative fluid fasting times and an earlier resumption of oral intake have helped in this respect. With longer and more complex procedures, nerve damage and other complications of adverse patient positions become more troublesome. Care should always be taken to ensure that the patient remains "comfortable" while unconscious. Finally, hospital-acquired infection remains a potential hazard which we must guard against with appropriate and effective measures.

1   Meyer-Witting M, Wilkinson DJ. A safe haven or a dangerous place–should we keep the anaesthetic room? (editorial) *Anaesthesia* 1992;**47**:1021–2.

2   Soni JC, Thomas DA. Comparison of anxiety before induction of anaesthesia in the anaesthetic room or operating theatre. *Anaesthesia* 1989;**44**:651–5.

3   Thompson N, Irwin MG, Gunawardene WMS, Chan L. Pre-operative parental anxiety. *Anaesthesia* 1996;**51**:1008–12.

4   Association of Anaesthetists of Great Britain and Ireland. *Recommendations for standards of monitoring during anaesthesia and recovery*, revised edition. London: AAGBI, 1994.

5   Gajraj RJ, Doi M, Mantzaridis H, Kenny GNC. Analysis of the EEG bispectrum, auditory evoked potentials and the EEG power spectrum during repeated transitions from consciousness to unconsciousness. *Br J Anaesth* 1998;**80**:46–52.

6   Leslie K, Sessler DI, Schroeder M, Walters K. Propofol blood concentration and the bispectral index predict suppression of learning during propofol/epidural anesthesia in volunteers. *Anesth Analg* 1995;**81**:1269–74.

7   Liu J, Singh H, White PF. Electroencephalographic bispectral index correlates with intra-operative recall and depth of propofol-induced sedation. *Anesth Analg* 1997;**84**:185–9.

8   Gan TJ, Glass PS, Windsor A *et al*. Bispectral index monitoring allows faster emergence and improved recovery from propofol, alfentanil, and nitrous oxide anesthesia. *Anesthesiology* 1997;**87**:808–15.

9   Song D, Joshi GP, White PF. Titration of volatile anesthetics using bispectral index facilitates recovery after ambulatory anesthesia. *Anesthesiology* 1997;**87**:842–8.

10   Thwaites AJ, Smith I. BIS during TCI propofol or sevoflurane anesthesia (abstract). *Anesthesiology* 1998;**89**:A899.

11   Obey PA, Ogg TW, Gilks WR. Temazepam and recovery in day surgery. *Anaesthesia* 1988;**43**:49–51.

12   Goldmann L, Ogg TW, Levey AB. Hypnosis and daycase anaesthesia. *Anaesthesia* 1988;**43**:466–9.

13   Tighe KE, Warner JA. The effect of co-induction with midazolam upon recovery from propofol infusion anaesthesia. *Anaesthesia* 1997;**52**:1000–4.

14   Djaiani G, Ribes-Pastor MP. Propofol auto-co-induction as an alternative to midazolam co-induction for ambulatory surgery. *Anaesthesia* 1999;**54**:63–7.

15. Hartung J. Twenty-four of twenty-seven studies show a greater incidence of emesis associated with nitrous oxide than with alternative anesthetics. *Anesth Analg* 1996;**83**:114–16.

16. Tramèr M, Moore A, McQuay H. Omitting nitrous oxide in general anaesthesia: meta-analysis of intraoperative awareness and postoperative emesis in randomized controlled trials. *Br J Anaesth* 1996;**76**:186–93.

17   Sukhani R, Lurie J, Jabamoni R. Propofol for ambulatory gynecological laparoscopy: does omission of nitrous oxide alter postoperative sequelae and recovery? *Anesth Analg* 1994;**78**:831–5.

18   Sengupta P, Plantevin OM. Nitrous oxide and day-case laparoscopy: effects on nausea, vomiting and return to normal activity. *Br J Anaesth* 1988;**60**:570–3.

19   Alcock R, Peachey T, Lynch M, McEwan T. Comparison of alfentanil with suxamethonium in facilitating nasotracheal intubation in day-case anaesthesia. *Br J Anaesth* 1993;**70**:34–7.

20   Thwaites AJ, Smith I. A double blind comparison of sevoflurane *versus* propofol and mivacurium for tracheal intubation in day case wisdom tooth extraction (abstract). *Br J Anaesth* 1998;**80**:A36.

21   Lepage J-Y, Malinovsky J-M, Malinge M *et al*. Pharmacodynamic dose-response and safety study of cisatracurium (51W89) in adult surgical patients during N_2O-O_2-opioid anesthesia. *Anesth Analg* 1996;**83**:823–9.

22   Kahwaji R, Bevan DR, Bikhazi G *et al*. Dose-ranging study in younger adult and elderly patients of Org 9487, a new, rapid-onset, short-duration muscle relaxant. *Anesth Analg* 1997;**84**:1011–18.

23   Ding Y, Fredman B, White PF. Use of mivacurium during laparoscopic surgery: effect of reversal drugs on postoperative recovery. *Anesth Analg* 1994;**78**:450–4.

24   Tramèr MR, Fuchs-Buder T. Omitting antagonism of neuromuscular block: effect on postoperative nausea and vomiting and risk of residual paralysis. A systematic review. *Br J Anaesth* 1999;**82**:379–86.

25 Baraka A, Yared J-P, Karam A-M, Winnie A. Glycopyrrolate-neostigmine and atropine-neostigmine mixtures affect postanesthetic arousal times differently. *Anesth Analg* 1980;**59**:431–4.

26 Verghese C, Brimacombe JR. Survey of laryngeal mask airway usage in 11910 patients: safety and efficacy for conventional and nonconventional usage. *Anesth Analg* 1996;**82**:129–33.

27 Verghese C, Smith TGC, Young E. Prospective survey of the use of the laryngeal mask airway in 2359 patients. *Anaesthesia* 1993;**48**:58–60.

28 Heijke SAM, Smith G, Key A. The effect of the Trendelenburg position on lower oesophageal sphincter tone. *Anaesthesia* 1991;**46**:185–7.

29 Chassard D, Berrada K, Tournadre J-P, Boulétreau P. The effects of neuromuscular block on peak airway pressure and abdominal elastance during pneumoperitoneum. *Anesth Analg* 1996;**82**:525–7.

30 Simpson RB, Russell D. Anaesthesia for daycase gynaecological laparoscopy: a survey of clinical practice in the United Kingdom. *Anaesthesia* 1999;**54**:72–6.

31 Goodwin APL, Rowe WL, Ogg TW. Day case laparoscopy. A comparison of two anaesthetic techniques using the laryngeal mask during spontaneous breathing. *Anaesthesia* 1992;**47**:892–5.

32 Swann DG, Spens H, Edwards SA, Chestnut RJ. Anaesthesia for gynaecological laparoscopy–a comparison between the laryngeal mask airway and tracheal intubation. *Anaesthesia* 1993;**48**:431–4.

33 Keane PW, Murray PF. Intravenous fluids in minor surgery. Their effect on recovery from anaesthesia. *Anaesthesia* 1986;**41**:635–7.

34 Yogendran S, Asokumar B, Cheng DCH, Chung F. A prospective randomized double-blind study of the effect of intravenous fluid therapy on adverse outcomes on outpatient surgery. *Anesth Analg* 1995;**80**:682–6.

35 Sessler DI. Mild perioperative hypothermia. *New Engl J Med* 1997;**336**:1730–7.

36 Leslie K, Sessler DI. Peri-operative hypothermia in the high-risk surgical patient. *Baillière's Clin Anaesthesiol* 1999;**13**(3):349–61.

37. Martin JT, Warner MA, eds. *Positioning in anesthesia and surgery*, 3rd edn. Philadelphia: WB Saunders, 1997.

38 Anon. Recommended practices: traffic patterns in the surgical suite. Association of Operating Room Nurses. *AORN Journal* 1993;**57**:730–4.

39 Gould D. Infection control in high-risk environments. *Nursing Standard* 1994;**8**:57–61.

40 Royal College of Anaesthetists and Association of Anaesthetists of Great Britain and Ireland. *Good practice. A guide for departments of anaesthesia.* London: RCA/AAGBI, 1998.

41 Brimacombe JR, Brain AIJ, Berry AM. *The laryngeal mask airway. A review and practical guide.* London: WB Saunders, 1997.

42 Ogg TW, Watson BJ. Aspects of day surgery and anaesthesia: a multidisciplinary approach. *Anaesthesia Rounds.* Cheshire: Zeneca Pharma, 1996.

3: Inhalation anaesthesia

ANGELA FRESCHINI, IAN SMITH

Overview

Inhalation anaesthesia has a long and established track record and, as such, will be familiar to most anaesthetists. The rapid expansion in day surgery coincided with the development of new anaesthetic drugs, both intravenous and inhaled. In recent years, however, many have gained the impression that inhalation anaesthesia is somewhat "old fashioned" and that intravenous anaesthesia is the only acceptable technique for day surgery. This is not the case, provided that inhaled anaesthetics are used appropriately.

There are undoubtedly disadvantages to inhalation anaesthesia in the day setting, but there are numerous benefits also. In many cases, intravenous anaesthesia does not produce significantly better outcome compared to inhalation anaesthesia, while the technique introduces unique problems of its own. Inhalation anaesthesia still represents the easiest way of achieving good intraoperative conditions without neuromuscular block, providing an excellent safeguard against intraoperative awareness. The inhaled anaesthetics remain simple to titrate against clinical signs, allowing rapid control over the depth of anaesthesia.

Newer inhaled anaesthetic drugs improve recovery times and enhance intraoperative control further. The "rediscovery" of inhalation induction in adults provides an interesting alternative anaesthetic technique which delivers some additional benefits, especially for very short cases. Perhaps even more important is a reevaluation of the need for some commonly used adjuvant drugs, especially opioid analgesics. As postoperative pain relief can now usually be provided by other means, it appears that the opioids do not improve our ability to deliver a satisfactory anaesthetic but may well contribute significantly to perioperative complications, especially postoperative nausea.

The aim of this chapter is to update readers on some of the newer inhaled anaesthetic agents and techniques and to encourage them to use these drugs in the optimal way, so as to achieve all the benefits of inhalation anaesthesia while reducing their disadvantages to a minimum.

Aims of day case anaesthesia

The ideal day case anaesthetic should allow rapid and smooth induction of anaesthesia, provide optimum surgical conditions, stable easily adjustable anaesthetic depth, adequate analgesia and amnesia, rapid and clear-headed recovery with residual analgesia and be associated with a low incidence of side effects, especially nausea and vomiting. Although no single agent fulfils all these criteria, the inhalation agents, in combination with appropriate non-opioid analgesics, are as effective as any other technique in achieving these aims.

A great many day case procedures remain straightforward cases of short duration with modest requirements for postoperative analgesia. For this common work, a simple and elegant anaesthetic technique, using as few drugs as possible, is an ideal approach. Day case surgery is also now expanding to accommodate procedures and patients previously managed in the inpatient setting. It would seem logical to use techniques which have been long established as safe and effective in this context, provided that they can be modified, by using shorter acting drugs, to achieve the additional requirements of day surgery.

Relative merits of inhalation anaesthesia

The major advantages and disadvantages of inhalation anaesthesia are shown in Box 3.1. The ubiquitous back-bar plus vaporiser ensures that this technique is easy to set up and use. It is a technique innate to all anaesthetists and therefore carries with it a strong history of safety. Its reliance on ventilatory variables automatically ensures impeccable airway management, which is essential however anaesthesia is delivered. The development of less irritant inhalants allows anaesthesia to be deepened rapidly, without inducing coughing or laryngospasm, which may otherwise compromise the airway.

Box 3.1 The relative merits of inhaled anaesthesia

Positive	*Negative*
• Easy to administer	• Drug delivery dependent upon
• Familiar	ventilatory characteristics
• Predictable intraoperative and	• Requirement for intraoperative and
recovery characteristics	recovery scavenging mechanisms
• Rapid induction and recovery	• Accepted higher incidence of PO
• Easily adjustable anaesthetic	than prop
depth	• May trigger malignant hyperpyr
• Invites low-flow anaesthesia	• Variable patient acceptance
• Anaesthetic depth monitored	inhalation induc
with end-tidal agent analysis	
• Recovery independent of	
metabolism	

PONV, postoperative nausea and vomiting

The proponents of intravenous IV anaesthesia claim improved recovery compared to inhalation anaesthesia. Recovery times are generally similar, or better, following inhalation anaesthesia compared to IV techniques, however, except when long-acting barbiturates are used for induction.[1] Intravenous (propofol) anaesthesia is also claimed to improve recovery times through a reduction in postoperative nausea and vomiting (PONV). While propofol does lower the incidence of PONV, this is predominantly an early effect and of negligible clinical benefit where the risk of PONV is relatively low.[2] Even where PONV is more likely, the effect of propofol is not clinically useful beyond the first few hours.[3] Delayed discharge resulting from PONV with inhalation-based anaesthetics is unusual,[4] even when these symptoms occur substantially more frequently compared to propofol.[5–7]

Table 3.1 Properties of the five currently available inhaled anaesthetic agents

	Halothane	Enflurane	Isoflurane	Desflurane	Sevoflurane
Introduced	1956	1971	1980	1993	1995
Blood gas solubility	2.5	1.9	1.4	0.42	0.69
MAC	0.75%	1.7%	1.15%	6%	2.05%
Induction characteristics	Smooth, slow, dysrhythmias common	Irritable	Irritable	Very irritable; not recommended	Smooth, rapid
Cardiac stability	Depressant, dysrhythmias common, sensitises heart to epinephrine	Depressant, some tachycardia	Depressant, some tachycardia	Mild depressant, stimulation with concentration increases	Mild depressant, normal heart rate
Ease of titration	Limited by solubility	Limited by potency	Limited by irritability	Limited by irritability	Easy
Recovery	Slow	Moderate	Moderate	Rapid	Rapid
Metabolism	≈20%	≈2%	≈0.2%	≈0.02%	≈5%

MAC, minimum alveolar concentration (in oxygen)

Inhalation anaesthetics provide a useful degree of muscle relaxation and will attenuate responses to moderate noxious stimuli. With nitrous oxide (N_2O), they can therefore be used as "single agents" during many minor and intermediate procedures. These properties can also supplement the effects of, and reduce the requirement for, adjunctive medications (e.g. opioid analgesics and neuromuscular blocking drugs) which may be required for more major day surgery operations. In contrast, propofol and all the other hypnotic components of total intravenous anaesthesia (TIVA) possess no intrinsic analgesic properties. Therefore separate provision for intraoperative analgesia must be made to facilitate a smooth maintenance period. It is difficult to control the depth of anaesthesia with IV anaesthesia and, whilst propofol has the most favourable properties for this, its complex pharmaco-kinetics still require the delivery rate to be adjusted frequently in order to maintain a particular plasma level. There is also a wide variation in patient response to a given plasma concentration and clinical signs are a less reliable guide to anaesthetic depth compared to volatile anaesthetics. It is therefore more difficult to prevent intraoperative movement or eliminate the risk of awareness (in the presence of neuromuscular block). Purposeful intraoper-ative movement is substantially more common during propofol anaesthesia compared to inhalational anaesthesia.[8] Propofol has also been shown to provide less satisfactory intraoperative conditions and require more intra-operative interventions than inhalational anaesthesia,[9] even when delivered by target-controlled infusion (TCI).[4]

Volatile anaesthetics are useful bronchodilators and may also provide a degree of cardioprotection.[10] These properties may be beneficial for those patients with more severe co-existing diseases who are now presenting for day surgery. As inpatients, this group has commonly been managed, to good effect, with inhaled anaesthetics; these should therefore be a good choice in the day care setting.

Inhalational anaesthetics have a significant economical advantage in that their consumption may be minimised by the use of low fresh gas flows. This can make their direct costs substantially lower than that of intravenously delivered anaesthesia. Although enthusiasts for IV anaesthesia argue that improvements in recovery times and side effects produce compensatory indirect savings,[11] the evidence is somewhat lacking. Many of these indirect costs are no more than estimates.[11] Even quite substantial reductions in recovery time (or even bypassing the recovery room completely) may have very little effect on staff costs[12] and any savings are highly dependent on employment methods. In any case, recovery times generally differ very little between inhalation and IV anaesthesia.[1] Even including the cost of PONV does not compensate for the substantially greater direct cost of IV anaesthesia.[6]

While no single agent can provide universally acceptable anaesthesia and analgesia, the inhalational agents provide all three components of the triad of hypnosis, analgesia and relaxation. Where this is insufficient, individual aspects can easily be supplemented, using a balanced approach. Recent developments in inhaled anaesthetics should ensure that these important drugs retain a prominent place in modern day case anaesthesia.

Choice of anaesthetic agents and technique

Induction

Until recently, day case anaesthesia was invariably induced with an IV bolus, irrespective of the maintenance anaesthetic technique. The advent of sevoflurane has made inhalation induction, in adults, a practical proposition.[13] This technique has a number of benefits (and some disadvantages), which will be considered in detail later. Inhalation induction has always had an important place in paediatric practice (see Chapter 9).

The most common day case anaesthetic technique probably remains a propofol bolus followed by an inhalation anaesthetic. Other IV induction agents all produce problems, including delayed recovery, excitement, venous irritation, PONV, and hallucinations. Propofol is therefore the drug of choice,[1] although it is far from ideal. Delivered as a manual bolus, propofol produces significant hypotension and apnoea, the latter of which can interfere with the introduction of the inhaled maintenance anaesthetic. Involuntary movements may occur and prevention of pain on injection requires the co-administration of substantial amounts of lidocaine (lignocaine). The ability to rapidly insert a laryngeal mask airway (LMA) with propofol has encouraged us to tolerate these significant disadvantages.

Delivering an inhaled anaesthetic following an IV bolus effectively involves a second induction, as adequate levels of the second drug must be achieved before the effects of the first agent wear off. This is especially important after short-acting induction agents such as propofol and in the unpremedicated anxious day case patient. By convention, however, the introduction of an inhalation anaesthetic after the patient is unconscious is defined as the start of maintenance.

Maintenance

We are currently presented with a choice of five inhalation anaesthetics which differ in solubility, potency, pungency, and side effect profile (Table 3.1). Solubility in blood is perhaps the most important property, as it determines the speed of induction and recovery. Solubility is somewhat analogous to volume of distribution; a more soluble drug requires a larger amount to be administered in order to achieve a given plasma concentration. As the rate of drug delivery is limited by alveolar ventilation, a requirement for more drug necessitates a longer period of administration. Eliminating the larger volume of the more soluble drug will also delay recovery; anaesthetics of low solubility are therefore desirable. Halothane and enflurane are the most soluble, sevoflurane and desflurane the least.

The pungency of the inhalation anaesthetic is also important. All volatile anaesthetics have a strong smell but some are more unpleasant than others. The more pungent agents may induce coughing, breath holding, and laryngospasm if inspired at high concentration. This may limit the ability to deepen anaesthesia rapidly, especially in patients with airway diseases. Airway irritation may also induce a hypertensive response to the more pungent anaesthetics.[14] Sevoflurane and halothane are the least pungent inhaled anaesthetics,[15] while isoflurane and desflurane are the most irritant.

The inhalation anaesthetics differ in potency, although this is relatively unimportant during the maintenance phase. Their general range of properties is similar, although there are minor differences between the various agents.

Halothane

Halothane is the most soluble of the inhalation anaesthetics, so slow recovery makes it an irrational choice for day surgery. In addition, halothane produces more dysrhythmias than other agents and concerns over its potential toxicity have greatly limited its use. Halothane has not been objectively studied as an adult day case anaesthetic in many years and is rarely used for this purpose. The excellent bronchodilation produced by halothane may be achieved just as well with sevoflurane.[16]

Enflurane

The first of the fluorinated methyl ethers to enter clinical practice, enflurane was once quite popular for day surgery. Despite its relatively high solubility, emergence and recovery times from enflurane anaesthesia are comparable to those achieved with an infusion of propofol.[17] The low potency of enflurane, combined with its solubility, limit the ability to achieve deep anaesthesia rapidly. Enflurane depresses respiration more than other fluorinated agents. In the spontaneously breathing patient, an adequate level of anaesthesia may not be achieved without significant hypercapnia. Enflurane also depresses cardiac output, produces seizure activity and is contraindicated in epileptic patients.

Although an adequate day case anaesthetic, enflurane offers no advantage over isoflurane and is now little used.

Isoflurane

With the decline in halothane use, isoflurane has become the "standard" inhaled anaesthetic against which others are compared. Isoflurane has intermediate solubility, with a blood:gas partition coefficient of 1.4. When used as a maintenance anaesthetic after induction with propofol, early recovery was similar, or only marginally impaired, compared to infusions of propofol,[1] while later recovery times did not differ. An advantage of propofol was only demonstrated after relatively long day case procedures.[18]

Isoflurane produces vasodilation and a reflex tachycardia. It causes only modest respiratory depression but is quite irritant to the airway. Caution is required when deepening anaesthesia rapidly in spontaneously breathing patients. Recent competition has made isoflurane very inexpensive, at least in the United Kingdom. It may be considered an acceptable, if somewhat basic, day case anaesthetic.

Desflurane

Desflurane *should* be an ideal day case anaesthetic. It has the lowest solubility of all available inhalation agents (blood:gas solubility coefficient 0.42) and is also the most metabolically stable. This latter feature is probably of no clinical significance in day case practice, however. The low solubility of desflurane initially caused it to be evaluated for inhalation induction, although it was abandoned as far too irritant for this purpose. Fortunately, respiratory irritation does not appear to be a major problem during the maintenance phase, even in patients breathing spontaneously through a LMA.[8] Rapid increases in desflurane anaesthesia should be avoided, however, as this can produce marked cardiovascular stimulation.[14]

Preliminary evaluations of desflurane suggested improved early recovery compared to isoflurane.[19, 20] Later recovery did not differ, however, and subsequent evaluation has suggested that there are only minor clinically important differences between desflurane and isoflurane or propofol" with respect to recovery times.[21] With the development of the concept of fast-track recovery (see Chapter 8), earlier emergence becomes more important and desflurane is able to achieve a higher proportion of "fast-track eligible" patients than either sevoflurane or propofol.[22] Desflurane may also prove useful as the duration of day surgery procedures increases; its low solubility ensures that recovery times are relatively unaffected by the duration of anaesthesia. Nevertheless, at present in the UK, desflurane is very little used for day surgery. This may be due to lingering concerns about its airway irritability, an unfamiliar dosage range and a tendency to cause more PONV compared to isoflurane.[23]

Sevoflurane

Sevoflurane (blood:gas partition coefficient 0.69) is substantially less soluble than isoflurane but more soluble than desflurane. It is the least pungent of all the inhaled anaesthetics and is well tolerated, even at high inspired concentrations. Sevoflurane causes minimal cardiac depression and does not produce tachycardia. These features, together with rapid recovery, allow the properties of muscle relaxation and potentiation of neuromuscular blocking drugs, which it shares with other inhaled anaesthetics, to be exploited to a greater degree.

Early recovery times following sevoflurane anaesthesia are significantly faster compared to isoflurane.[24] Emergence may be slightly faster[7, 22] or similar compared to propofol[5] and similar[22, 25] or slightly slower compared to desflurane.[26] Intermediate recovery and discharge times appear comparable for all these techniques, however. A large multicentre trial has shown that, compared to isoflurane, maintenance of anaesthesia with sevoflurane results in significantly less nausea.[24]

Inhalation induction

Inhalation induction is *possible* with any of the available volatile anaesthetics. Until recently, however, this approach was unpopular with patients because the process was too slow and the available drugs too pungent. Nevertheless, inhalation induction is a long-established technique with a tradition of safety and the potential to offer several benefits.

Low solubility inhaled anaesthetics, such as cyclopropane, were once popular for day case anaesthesia because they facilitated rapid recovery. These drugs were ultimately abandoned because of their explosive potential. The arrival of desflurane, with a similar solubility to cyclopropane, reawakened interest in inhalation induction in day cases. While desflurane could induce anaesthesia rapidly (and improve awakening compared to propofol induction), it proved too pungent and irritant to be practically useful.[27] In contrast, sevoflurane proved more useful because it combined reasonably low solubility with low pungency, allowing high concentrations to be inspired to facilitate induction.[13, 28]

When anaesthesia was induced with a tidal breathing technique, in which 8% sevoflurane was delivered from the outset, the induction process was clinically indistinguishable (by a blinded observer) to that achieved with propofol, despite somewhat longer induction times in the inhalation group.[13] The majority of patients found inhalation induction acceptable, although a minority did not. Our subsequent clinical experience, however, suggests that outside the constraints of a clinical trial, inhalation induction with sevoflurane is generally well received. Faster induction times have been reported using a vital capacity induction technique,[29] in some cases achieving more rapid induction than IV propofol. In a randomised comparison, however, Baker and Smith found no difference in induction times between tidal breathing and vital capacity techniques.[30] This may be due to poor patient compliance and/or a loose fitting mask with the vital capacity technique, which would limit its effectiveness. In any case, the average day case anaesthetist is likely to feel more comfortable using the more familiar tidal ventilation technique. This can only increase patient safety.

Whatever technique is used, sevoflurane should be introduced at 8% initially. Slow, step-wise increases in sevoflurane concentration during induction produce more excitatory phenomena and delay loss of consciousness.[31] Furthermore, this technique is unnecessary with sevoflurane, as high initial inspired concentrations produce few respiratory effects.[13]

The VIMA concept: advantages and disadvantages

Given the frequency with which inhalation agents are used to maintain day case anaesthesia, the adoption of inhalation induction allows the use of the same agent for induction and maintenance. This should eliminate the transition from IV induction agent to inhaled maintenance drug and result in a smoother period of anaesthesia following induction. Clinical observation and some preliminary clinical evidence[13] appear to support this notion. This approach was initially described as "single-agent anaesthesia", a term which was confusing due to the co-administration of N_2O and sometimes other adjuvants. Consequently, the acronym VIMA (Volatile Induction and Maintenance of Anaesthesia) was devised.

In addition to avoiding the problem of a transition between two different types of drug, VIMA offers several other clinical advantages. In particular, a number of the disadvantages of the IV induction drug are avoided. These include a reduction in the duration and magnitude of the hypotension associated with manually delivered propofol.[13] Apnoea is virtually eliminated, ensuring that anaesthesia and oxygen continue to be delivered. Although apnoea can be managed easily, it does tend to further complicate the transition from IV induction to inhalation maintenance. In addition, respiratory rate and pattern are retained as clinical monitors, while the anaesthetist's hands are free for tasks other than squeezing the reservoir bag. Finally, inhalation induction offers a painless option for needle phobics, a condition reported to affect at least 10% of the population.[32] Inhalation induction with sevoflurane does not appear to induce significant complications, such as laryngospasm, so it should be safe to defer IV cannulation until loss of consciousness (a common practice in paediatric anaesthesia). Access should of course be established as soon as possible after loss of consciousness, for obvious safety reasons. This should ideally be achieved before instrumenting the airway or performing any other interventions which might provoke laryngospasm.

Elimination of an IV induction agent may also affect early recovery. Awakening after sevoflurane VIMA occurred significantly earlier compared to propofol induction followed by sevoflurane maintenance lasting 10[13] to 20[33] minutes. The difference in time was only a couple of minutes, although this may be an important difference after short-duration, high turnover procedures, especially when fast-track recovery is intended. This residual sedative effect of propofol induction is not apparent when the duration of anaesthesia approaches 30 minutes, however.[34]

An inhalation induction with sevoflurane provides acceptable conditions for LMA insertion and also for tracheal intubation. Although many day case procedures are performed with the LMA (Chapter 2), tracheal intubation may still be required on occasions. Using a technique which eliminates neuromuscular block allows light anaesthesia to be used (to facilitate rapid recovery) without the risk of intraoperative awareness; if anaesthesia becomes too light, the patient will move. Tracheal intubation may be performed after inhaling 8% sevoflurane for approximately four minutes in adults[35] and 2.5 minutes in children.[36] At these times, tracheal intubating conditions were comparable to propofol-mivacurium and propofol-succinylcholine, respectively. Tracheal intubation can also be achieved using IV drugs without neuromuscular block, although comparative studies with VIMA have not been conducted.

VIMA is not a perfect technique and is associated with a few problems. The possibility that inhalation induction results in unacceptable levels of operating room pollution seems to have been discounted.[37] Although most studies have shown inhalation induction to be well tolerated, it is probably still not as acceptable as the familiar IV induction. This may be because of residual memories from previous gaseous induction drugs, poor technique or simply a dislike of the smell of sevoflurane. In contrast, some patients definitely prefer an inhaled induction and this is not just confined to needle phobics. Allowing the patient some choice in their induction seems the best approach.

Several studies have shown significant levels of PONV after VIMA compared to propofol anaesthesia.[4, 6] This may be an inherent problem with the technique, caused either by the inhaled induction or, more likely, by the elimination of propofol. The effect of opioid analgesics must also be considered, however. Comparative studies with propofol anaesthesia have co-administered fentanyl with VIMA. For most current day case procedures, intraoperative opioids are not necessary; the inhaled anaesthetic can blunt responses to surgery, while non-opioid analgesics (Chapter 7) can take care of postoperative pain. In the absence of opioids, it is our experience that VIMA is associated with a far lower, and clinically acceptable, level of PONV.[38] This feature of VIMA may limit its applicability for more major day surgery procedures, where opioids are required, although the effects of prophylactic antiemetics have not yet been fully evaluated.

From a cost-effectiveness point of view, VIMA represents the most efficient way of delivering sevoflurane and is less expensive during both induction and maintenance compared to propofol-sevoflurane or propofol anaesthesia.[6] If PONV is problematic, however, this may negate some of the cost advantage.

Administration of inhalation anaesthetics

The delivery of inhaled anaesthetics requires a similar understanding of basic pharmacokinetic principles, such as early redistribution, intercompartment transfer and elimination, to those which apply to IV drugs. Furthermore, the situation is complicated by the addition of two extra compartments, the breathing circuit and the lungs, interposed between the point of drug delivery and its effect. Nevertheless, most anaesthetists will be familiar with titrating inhalation anaesthetics. In the absence of a perfect monitor of anaesthetic depth, clinical signs, especially respiratory rate and pattern, give a reasonable guide to the adequacy of inhalation anaesthesia.

Drug titration is aided by the widespread availability of end-expired agent monitoring. This gives an indication that the level of anaesthesia is in approximately the correct range and, most importantly, confirms that drug is actually being delivered.

In titrating inhalation anaesthetics, the MAC value may be of some use. Two important facts must be remembered, however. First, MAC defines the alveolar concentration which prevents movement in just half the subjects; there is considerable interpatient variability in MAC. Secondly, although MAC defines an alveolar concentration, prevention of response actually requires a given concentration at the site of anaesthetic effect. There is always a delay in equilibration between plasma (alveolar) and effect site concentrations. Therefore, a given end-expired concentration will not be reflected in the effect site early in anaesthetic delivery or soon after a change in delivered concentration. This explains why patients may respond, especially at the initial incision, despite an apparently adequate measured anaesthetic concentration.

Low-flow anaesthesia

The advantages of low-flow anaesthesia are well known and include retention of heat and moisture, similar efficiency with spontaneous or controlled ventilation, reduced environmental pollution, and savings in inhaled anaesthetic costs. It is a common belief that day case procedures are too brief to benefit from low-flow anaesthesia, but this is not true. For example, Logan showed that reducing gas flows from 3 to 1 l/min produced a 34% saving in enflurane consumption during cases lasting approximately 11 minutes.[39] Low solubility anaesthetics permit earlier reduction in fresh gas flow. It has been suggested that flows may be reduced after about four minutes using desflurane and eight minutes with sevoflurane.[40] Mapleson calculated that gas flows could be reduced even earlier (at one minute for desflurane or sevoflurane), if a maximum concentration of the inhaled anaesthetic is delivered until the desired end-expired value is achieved and assuming adequate preoxygenation.[41] In practice, fresh gas flow may be reduced to 1 l/min immediately after LMA insertion following an inhalation induction, although this economic benefit is only possible if the same breathing circuit can be used throughout induction and maintenance.

Low-flow anaesthesia is made simple and safe by oxygen and expired agent concentration monitoring. Even if complete equilibration and/or denitrogenation have not been achieved, compensatory adjustments may be made to the fresh gas mixture.

Hazards of low-flow anaesthesia
Interactions between inhaled anaesthetics and carbon dioxide adsorbents may produce potentially toxic products. This is rarely a problem in practice,

however. Several inhaled anaesthetics can produce carbon monoxide in the presence of exceedingly dry soda lime (and especially baralyme). While this may result in patient harm, soda lime is unlikely to become sufficiently dry under normal conditions of use. Sevoflurane breaks down to compound A in the presence of soda lime. The levels produced are low and significant clinical harm has not been observed, even under extreme conditions. Even in the United States, where very conservative fresh gas flow rate restrictions were in place, these have now been relaxed to permit the delivery of 1 MAC sevoflurane for two hours at 1 l/min flows. This should be sufficient for most day surgery procedures. Most of Europe (and the rest of the world) places no flow restrictions on sevoflurane.

Concomitant agents

Nitrous oxide

Nitrous oxide (N_2O) is a potent analgesic; inhalation of 20–50% mixtures in oxygen may have similar effects to standard doses of morphine.[42] Since both onset and offset of analgesia are extremely rapid it would seem that this agent would be the ideal intraoperative anaesthetic adjuvant. However, N_2O is theoretically an emetic and it is generally believed to be associated with postoperative nausea and vomiting. The reason for its emetic potential is as yet not clearly determined, although diffusion into closed cavities such as the middle ear (where it causes changes of pressure) and the gut (which causes distension) are the most likely factors. Other implicated factors include activation of receptors within the medullary dopaminergic system, stimulation of the sympathetic nervous system and activation of opioid receptors within the central nervous system. Although N_2O is one of the many causes of PONV, its effect is relatively small in practice,[3] especially when weighed against the need to prevent intraoperative awareness[43] and to provide alternative (usually opioid) forms of analgesia.

Opioid analgesics

It is common practice to administer small doses of opioid analgesics, usually combined with the induction dose of propofol, as a supplement to inhalation anaesthesia. This practice has a number of advantages.

- Small reduction in propofol induction dose.
- Reduced response to insertion of LMA.
- Provision of intraoperative analgesia (reduces haemodynamic and somatic response to surgery).

It is a common belief that opioid supplementation will also enhance early postoperative analgesia. There is little evidence to support this notion, however, especially when short-acting opioids (e.g. fentanyl, alfentanil, remifentanil) are used. In addition, the use of supplemental opioids has several disadvantages.

- Prolonged apnoea and respiratory depression.
- Delayed recovery due to sedation.
- Postoperative nausea and vomiting.

Even the use of quite modest doses of opioid analgesics can substantially increase the incidence of PONV, with much of the effect occurring after the patient is discharged home.[44] Within the day care setting, it would seem sensible to avoid the administration of any opioid, whenever possible, and provide postoperative analgesia with local anaesthesia and NSAIDs. Compared to fentanyl, NSAIDs provide substantially better and more prolonged postoperative analgesia[45, 46] with a lower incidence of PONV. Increasing the volatile anaesthetic concentration slightly can usually suppress most intraoperative responses to surgery; the VIMA technique achieves this particularly well. Administering the local anaesthetic before the incision or in the early intraoperative period will also help.

Opioid analgesia may occasionally be required for more stressful procedures where anaesthesia alone cannot control intraoperative responses. Any of the short-acting opioids may be used. Alfentanil and remifentanil both have the advantage of a rapid onset of action, but they cause more respiratory depression than fentanyl. It is particularly difficult to find a dose of remifentanil which is effective yet permits spontaneous ventilation to continue in combination with inhalation anaesthesia.[47] There is little evidence that alfentanil and remifentanil provoke any less PONV than fentanyl, although all three are preferable to morphine, which also produces prolonged postoperative sedation.

Recovery

As already discussed, rapid recovery will be facilitated by the selection of low solubility anaesthetics. Because the blood flow through the lungs is so great, metabolism of inhaled anaesthetics is unimportant in their speed of elimination. Recovery is predominantly related to solubility in blood, although solubility in other body tissues will also increase uptake and delay recovery. Transfer to these tissues takes some time, however, and differences in tissue solubility are less important in determining recovery times in short day case procedures than they are in longer cases.

In addition to solubility, the titration and conduct of anaesthesia will affect recovery. Anaesthesia will need to be relatively deep at the beginning of surgery and at other periods of major stimulus, but may be allowed to lighten somewhat towards the end of the procedure. The end-expired agent concentration provides a guide but clinical signs and experience are more important. Changes in respiratory rate or pattern, heart rate and blood pressure or patient movement all indicate that anaesthesia is inadequate. Much greater caution will be required in the presence of neuromuscular block. Titration of anaesthesia with the aid of the bispectral index (BIS) monitor (see Chapter 2) has been shown to reduce inhaled anaesthetic consumption and shorten recovery times.[48] There is considerable interpatient variability in BIS values, however. In addition, BIS neither predicts patient movement nor correlates with recovery times.[49] Therefore, using BIS as a guide to delivering the barest minimum of anaesthesia should only be attempted with extreme caution, especially in the presence of neuromuscular block.

The rate of recovery will also be dependent upon the combined effects of all the drugs administered, as with IV. anaesthesia. As N_2O has low blood solubility, delivering approximately half of the anaesthesia with N_2O while the remainder is provided by another insoluble anaesthetic should result in more rapid recovery than if a single drug is used (in higher dose) to provide the whole anaesthetic. In the former case, recovery will occur along two almost parallel drug elimination slopes. In the latter case, there will be a single recovery curve, of similar slope but commencing at a greater height; recovery should therefore take longer. There is some evidence to support this notion.[50]

Practicalities of inhalation anaesthesia

Overpressure

Overpressure is a familiar concept in inhalation anaesthesia, although it is now being applied with IV anaesthesia (see Chapter 4). Overpressure involves delivering a higher concentration of anaesthetic than that required, in order to produce a high concentration gradient and speed the achievement of a desired alveolar (blood) concentration. Overpressure may be used at induction of anaesthesia, at the commencement of an inhaled maintenance anaesthetic following IV induction or whenever it is desired to increase the depth of anaesthesia rapidly.

The ability to tolerate overpresure will vary for different anaesthetics. For irritant agents (e.g. isoflurane, desflurane), high concentrations may induce coughing, laryngospasm or cardiovascular stimulation. For all agents, overpressure will induce hypotension and respiratory depression if it is not removed once the desired concentration is achieved. However, it may be possible to retain a moderate degree of overpressure in order to increase the brain concentration once an effective alveolar concentration has been achieved. The brain concentration will always lag behind changes in alveolar concentration due to the phenomenon of effect site delay. This may be observed, for example, during an inhalation induction with sevoflurane. By the time adequate conditions for LMA insertion have been achieved, the end-expired sevoflurane concentration typically reads between 3–4%. This is substantially higher than the 1.1–1.4% necessary during the maintenance phase (assuming the use of N_2O). The discrepancy is due to the delay in equilibration between sevoflurane in the blood and at its site(s) of action. If the same circle absorber breathing circuit can be used throughout the whole case (i.e. no separate anaesthetic induction room), the fresh gas flow may be reduced immediately to 1 l/min (or lower) and the vaporiser turned off. The end-expired sevoflurane concentration will gradually decrease as further redistribution occurs. The vaporiser will not need to be turned back on again until the alveolar concentration declines to an appropriate mainte-nance level or the patient demonstrates signs of light anaesthesia.

A similar approach may be used with other inhaled anaesthetics whenever a rapid increase in delivered anaesthetic concentration produces an "overshoot" in end-expired concentration. Exactly the same suspension of drug delivery occurs (automatically) when the target propofol concen-tration is reduced on a TCI delivery system (see Chapter 4). It is possible that the prolonged elevated end-expired concentration may produce moderate hypotension, although in practice this appears well tolerated, especially with sevoflurane. This technique has the advantage of main-taining relatively deep anaesthesia during the early part of surgery, where the stimulus is greatest, while facilitating a reduction in anaesthetic depth in anticipation of the end of the procedure.

Suggested practical techniques

Anaesthesia techniques will vary slightly depending upon the nature of the procedure, several patient factors, and the method of airway management. In addition, most practitioners will have their own selection of techniques which have served them well over the years. The following are offered as suggestions to the novice or to the experienced practitioner to evaluate against their existing practice.

Intravenous bolus, inhaled maintenance

The induction dose of propofol in fit, unpremedicated day cases may be 2.5–3 mg/kg or even more. Delivering the propofol slowly, titrated against loss of verbal contact, will reduce the induction dose somewhat and also reduce complications. Administering midazolam 1–2 mg about two minutes before induction will substantially reduce the propofol dose without dramatically delaying recovery. Alternatively, administering 20–30 mg of propofol prior to the main induction dose will have a somewhat similar effect.[51]

In most cases, adequate jaw relaxation for LMA insertion will be achieved within 60 seconds. If not, the maintenance vapour may be introduced by mask. Fentanyl 50–100 μg or alfentanil 0.5–1 mg will minimise coughing on LMA insertion and reduce intraoperative responsiveness. However, this same act will prolong apnoea, substantially increase the incidence of PONV and will make no difference to early postoperative analgesia. We recommend that supplemental opioids are only administered if really necessary.

The maintenance anaesthetic should be introduced starting with 1.5% isoflurane, 7.5% desflurane or 2.5% sevoflurane delivered in N_2O 4 l/min and O_2 2 l/min. Subsequent titration of anaesthetic delivery should be based on clinical signs, but is likely to result in the end-expired concentrations being in the range of 0.6–0.8%, 3–4%, and 1.0–1.4% for isoflurane, desflurane, and sevoflurane, respectively. If using a circle absorber system, the fresh gas flow may be reduced to 0.8–1 l/min (using a 50:50 mixture of O_2/N_2O) when the end-expired concentration reaches the desired value. This will result in a relatively early reduction in fresh gas flow and will probably require an increase in vaporiser setting to maintain that level following fresh gas flow reduction (as a result of continuing uptake). The reduction in flow more than compensates for the extra cost of a higher vaporiser setting, however. Remember that in the early stages of anaesthesia, an adequate end-expired concentration will not guarantee an adequate effect site concentration.

The use of low fresh gas flows means that changes in vaporiser setting will not immediately result in changes in anaesthetic depth. This greater "inertia" can make for a smoother maintenance phase. Changes in effect can still be made, either by a larger change in the vaporiser setting or by temporarily increasing the fresh gas flow until the desired change occurs. Vapours of low solubility provide a greater degree of control at low flow than do more soluble ones. If the end of surgery can be anticipated in advance, the vaporiser may be switched off and the inspired (and expired) vapour concentration allowed to decline slowly. The rate of decrease may be slowed further by also discontinuing N_2O and continuing at a low flow of oxygen. The low fresh gas flow prevents the blood anaesthetic concentration from decreasing too rapidly but allows the return of anaesthetic from peripheral sites to the central compartment to start, which hastens the subsequent recovery process. When surgery is finished, the oxygen flow is increased to 8–10 l/min to flush out the residual anaesthetic. In contrast, if the completion of surgery is delayed, vapour delivery may be recommenced at any point before anaesthesia becomes too light. This technique is summarised in Box 3.2.

VIMA

The VIMA technique is suitable for a wide range of day case procedures. It is most efficient where the same circle system can be used for induction and

Box 3.2 Summary of the intravenous bolus, inhaled maintenance technique (see text for more details)

Induction	• Midazolam 1–2 mg or propofol 20–30 mg • Wait 2 minutes • Propofol injected slowly until loss of verbal contact
At loss of consciousness	• Manually ventilate with N_2O 4 l/min O_2 2 l/min • Insert LMA if jaw relaxed • If jaw not relaxed, start maintenance anaesthetic
Maintenance	• Isoflurane: start at 1.5%, aim for 0.6–0.8% end-expired • Desflurane: start at 7.5%, aim for 3–4% end-expired • Sevoflurane: start at 2.5%, aim for 1.0–1.4% end-expired • Reduce gas flow to 0.8–1 l/min/ when "target" end-expired concentration achieved • Titrate delivered anaesthetic against clinical response • Aim for lower end-expired values towards end of case
Recovery	• Turn vaporiser and N_2O off before end of case • Be prepared to restart anaesthetic delivery if necessary • Flush circuit with O_2 8–10 l/min at end of case

maintenance (i.e. no anaesthetic induction room) and for very short procedures. Where circumstances dictate, it can also be used to facilitate spontaneous (and controlled) ventilation through an endotracheal tube. It is recommended to use a clear plastic mask and to use gentleness and friendly reassurance throughout induction (as for any anaesthetic). The tidal breathing technique (summarised in Box 3.3) works well in routine practice; a vital capacity technique may be selected in an especially cooperative patient or where a fast induction is especially desirable.

Preoxygenation may be performed, if desired, but is not really necessary as the patient will breathe a high oxygen concentration during induction. It may be advisable to let the patient hold the mask themselves, encouraging them to hold it as tight as is comfortable. Patients often hold the mask tighter than we would consider applying it ourselves! At the start of induction, set oxygen and N_2O flows of 2 l/min and 4 l/min, respectively and turn the sevoflurane vaporiser directly to 8%. Ask the patient to breathe deeply and reassure them that they will notice a sweet, fruity or minty smell. Check for obvious leaks and correct the mask fit as necessary. Continue talking to the patient, reassuring them and encouraging deep breathing.

Box 3.3 Summary of the volatile induction and maintenance of anaesthesia (VIMA) technique, using a tidal breathing induction method (see text for more details)

Induction	• Use clear mask, apply gently or allow patient to hold • Preoxygenate, if desired (usually unnecessary) • Start O_2 2 l/min, N_2O 4 l/min, sevoflurane 8% • Reassure patient about "sweet" or "fruity" smell • Check mask seal, encourage deep breathing • Check for loss of verbal contact
At loss of consciousness	• Assist ventilation by gentle bag compression • Insert LMA when jaw relaxed • Wait at least four minutes before tracheal intubation

Maintenance	• If using circle system from outset:
	  • reduce gas flow to 0.8–1 l/min immediately after LMA insertion/intubation and turn vaporiser off
	  • observe patient and end-expired concentration
	  • restart sevoflurane when end-tidal ≤1.2% or at first signs of "light" anaesthesia
	• With separate induction room:
	  • reduce vaporiser to 2–3%
	  • reduce gas flow to 0.8–1 l/min 2–3 minutes after transfer to circle system
	  • titrate sevoflurane against clinical response
	• Use 8% "bolus" to rapidly deepen anaesthesia
	• Turn vaporiser off in event of end-expired "overshoot"

Recovery	• As Box 3.2

Some patients experience mild euphoria just before loss of consciousness. Once the patient becomes unresponsive, begin to support their breathing by gentle bag compression. It is not necessary to take over breathing completely, but desirable to maintain a good tidal volume as anaesthetic-induced respiratory depression progresses. The LMA may be inserted as soon as the jaw is relaxed. This typically takes about 2.5–3 minutes. If tracheal intubation is desired, continue with 8% sevoflurane until at least four minutes from the start of induction. If coughing or excitement does occur, which is rare, continue to deepen anaesthesia with 8% sevoflurane until the condition resolves. Do not attempt intubation or LMA insertion if the patient is not settled.

If anaesthesia is induced in the operating theatre, the fresh gas flow may be reduced to 1 l/min and the vaporiser turned off immediately after LMA insertion. If a separate anaesthetic induction room has been used, reduce the vaporiser to 2–3% and then reduce gas flows within about two minutes of changing to a circle system in the operating room. If the gas flow is reduced immediately after LMA insertion, the end-expired sevoflurane concentration will be seen to be in the range 3–4%, which is much higher than the required maintenance level and the result of effect site delay. At 1 l/min, it may be 10–15 minutes before anaesthetic delivery has to restart. In contrast, if it is necessary to deepen anaesthesia at any time, the vaporiser may be opened directly to 8%. This "inhaled bolus" will be well tolerated and usually produces a reasonably rapid response. It should only be necessary to increase the fresh gas flow if the patient was exceptionally "light". Again, because of effect site delay, there will usually be some over-shoot in end-expired (or plasma) anaesthetic level. Consequently, the vaporiser may again be turned off until an appropriate level is achieved. This "saw-tooth" anaesthesia *delivery* pattern is greatly smoothed by the low fresh gas flow and can result in a stable and very economic anaesthetic.

Because opioids appear to significantly increase PONV in association with VIMA, they should only be used if intraoperative patient responses cannot be adequately controlled by increasing the vapour concentration and should not be given routinely. If the technique outlined above is used, intraoperative opioids will rarely be found to be necessary.

Vital capacity induction

This technique is summarised in Box 3.4. Vital capacity induction requires a breathing circuit with a bag of at least 4 litres capacity (although a pair of 2 litre bags may be connected by a Y-piece). The circuit should be primed with 8% sevoflurane in N_2O 4 l/min and O_2 2 l/min until the bag is reasonably full. This can be achieved by manually occluding the outlet of the angle piece from the inside of the patient mask. There is no need to prime the expiratory limb of the breathing circuit or to cause excessive distension of the bag; excess gas will simply be lost to atmosphere when the occlusion is removed. While priming the circuit, the patient can be given (or reminded of) their instructions. They should be told to breathe out as far as possible, at which point the mask (attached to the primed circuit) is tightly applied. The patient is then asked to take as big a breath as possible and to hold this for as long as they can. Care should be taken to ensure a good seal during the vital capacity breath, to prevent air dilution. The patient should be encouraged to keep breathing in during the first breath to ensure maximum volume. With a good seal and correct technique, loss of consciousness within 20–40 seconds is possible but many patients require longer than this, especially when subsequent breaths are taken. Once unconsciousness is achieved, the remainder of the technique is the same as for the tidal breathing approach.

Box 3.4 Summary of the vital capacity inhaled induction technique (see text for more details)

Preparation and priming	• Use breathing system with 4 litre bag • Occlude patient end of breathing circuit • Start O_2 2 l/min, N_2O 4 l/min, sevoflurane 8% • Allow bag to fill for 30–45 seconds • Instruct patient in technique during priming (or before)
Induction	• Have patient breathe out as far as possible • Apply mask (attached to primed circuit) to patient • Check for good seal, ensure no leak • Ask patient to breathe in as far as possible • Encourage patient to hold breath as long as possible • Allow further breaths, if necessary • Check for loss of verbal contact
At loss of consciousness	• As Box 3.2

Future developments

Even the most recently introduced inhaled anaesthetics were synthesised many years ago. All the other molecules in the families of the existing anaesthetics have been synthesised and screened. It is quite unlikely that any volatile compound with anaesthetic properties that is not toxic or too unstable has been overlooked. In addition, any new inhaled anaesthetic would have to offer very significant advantages over existing agents to be commercially successful. At present, no new volatile anaesthetic drugs are expected to be introduced.

There is one remaining, known inhaled anaesthetic, the noble gas xenon. Xenon has a MAC value of 71% and is very insoluble, with a blood:gas partition coefficient of 0.14.[52] Induction with xenon is very rapid, although limited by the inability to deliver significant overpressure due to the high MAC value. Recovery is also rapid, faster than that which can be achieved with isoflurane or sevoflurane.[53] In addition, the effects of xenon on other organ systems seem relatively benign. Unfortunately, xenon is extremely expensive, at least 10 times that of existing anaesthetics. The finite reserves of xenon, coupled with increased use in the space industry,[52] mean that the price is unlikely to decrease in the foreseeable future. Although xenon may be a promising future day case anaesthetic, it seems unlikely to enter routine clinical practice at present.

Summary

Although induction of anaesthesia with intravenous anaesthetics is commonplace, so too is the use of inhaled anaesthetics for maintenance. Although this approach involves a transition from one type of drug to another, it has worked well in a variety of settings for a long time. The benefits of inhaled anaesthesia during the maintenance phase have generally been so great that the inconvenience of the transition has been tolerated.

Improvements in inhaled anaesthetics have resulted in faster recovery and even better intraoperative control. Inhaled anaesthetics produce reasonably predictable effects on clinical signs and the ability to measure these agents in breath provides reassurance that an approximately adequate amount is being delivered. Sevoflurane, with its minimal airway irritation and comparatively benign cardiovascular effects, has made control of anaesthesia even easier. In addition, it has made inhalation induction a practical and beneficial proposition, allowing that awkward transition to be eliminated, while still retaining the benefits of inhalation anaesthetics during maintenance.

Most inhaled anaesthetics, combined with nitrous oxide, are sufficiently "complete" anaesthetics that additional adjuvants are unnecessary. This results in a simplified technique but also provides advantages. The elimination of neuromuscular block retains respiratory characteristics as a useful monitor and safeguards against awareness. The elimination of opioid analgesics reduces PONV, one of the major drawbacks of inhaled anaesthesia, to levels which are usually acceptable. Finally, inhalation anaesthesia is economical, especially when using low fresh gas flows, provided that postoperative nausea can be minimised as described.

Induction of anaesthesia with any of the schemes described in detail will be rapid, safe, and controlled and will permit surgery to commence promptly. Unwanted movement during surgery will be uncommon, especially using the VIMA technique, which ensures deep anaesthesia at the early, more stimulating phase. Recovery from these regimens will be rapid, provided that care is taken not to provide excessively deep anaesthesia in the final moments of the operation. If postoperative analgesia is provided with appropriately timed and adequate doses of NSAIDs and local anaesthesia, patients will awaken in comfort and with a low incidence of PONV. In addition, with the shorter acting drugs, patients will be clear-headed and ready for early hospital discharge.

Clearly other techniques are also suitable for day case surgery but inhaled anaesthesia has stood the test of time and still has much to offer.

1   Smith I, White PF, Nathanson M, Gouldson R. Propofol: an update on its clinical use. *Anesthesiology* 1994;**81**:1005–43.

2   Tramèr M, Moore A, McQuay H. Propofol anaesthesia and postoperative nausea and vomiting: quantitative systemic review of randomized controlled studies. *Br J Anaesth* 1997;**78**:247–55.

3   Tramèr M, Moore A, McQuay H. Meta-analytic comparison of prophylactic antiemetic efficacy for postoperative nausea and vomiting: propofol anaesthesia *vs* omitting nitrous oxide *vs* total i.v. anaesthesia with propofol. *Br J Anaesth* 1997;**78**:256–9.

4   Smith I, Thwaites AJ. Target-controlled propofol *vs.* sevoflurane: a double-blind, randomised comparison in day-case anaesthesia. *Anaesthesia* 1999;**54**:745–52.

5   Fredman B, Nathanson MH, Smith I, Wang J, Klein K, White PF. Sevoflurane for outpatient anesthesia: a comparison with propofol. *Anesth Analg* 1995;**81**:823–8.

6   Smith I, Terhoeve PA, Hennart D *et al.* A multicentre comparison of the costs of anaesthesia with sevoflurane or propofol. *Br J Anaesth* 1999;**83**:564–70.

7   Ræder JC, Gupta A, Pedersen FM. Recovery characteristics of sevoflurane- or propofol-based anaesthesia for day-surgery. *Acta Anaesthesiol Scand* 1997;**41**:988–94.

8   Ashworth J, Smith I. Comparison of desflurane with isoflurane or propofol in spontaneously breathing ambulatory patients. *Anesth Analg* 1998;**87**:312–18.

9   DeGrood PMRM, Harbers JBM, van Egmond J, Crul JF. Anaesthesia for laparoscopy. A comparison of five techniques including propofol, etomidate, thiopentone and isoflurane. *Anaesthesia* 1987;**42**:815–23.

10   Lynch C III. Anaesthetic preconditioning. Not just for the heart? (editorial) *Anesthesiology* 1999;**91**:606-8

11   Rowe WL. Economics and anaesthesia. *Anaesthesia* 1998;**53**:782–8.

12   Dexter F, Macario A, Manberg PJ, Lubarsky DA. Computer simulation to determine how rapid anesthetic recovery protocols to decrease the time for emergence or increase the Phase I Postanesthesia care unit bypass rate affect staffing of an ambulatory surgery center. *Anesth Analg* 1999;**88**:1053–63.

13   Thwaites A, Edmends S, Smith I. Inhalation induction with sevoflurane–a double-blind comparison with propofol. *Br J Anaesth* 1997;**78**:356–61.

14   Weiskopf RB, Eger EI II, Daniel M, Noorani M. Cardiovascular stimulation induced by rapid increases in desflurane concentration in humans results from activation of tracheopulmonary and systemic receptors. *Anesthesiology* 1995;**83**:1171–8.

15   Doi M, Ikeda K. Airway irritation produced by volatile anaesthetics during brief inhalation: comparison of halothane, enflurane, isoflurane and sevoflurane. *Can J Anaesth* 1993;**40**:122–6.

16   Rooke GA, Choi J-H, Bishop MJ. The effect of isoflurane, halothane, servoflurane, and thiopental/nitrous oxide on respiratory system resistance after tracheal intubation. *Anaesthesiology* 1997;**86**:1294–9.

17   Ding Y, Fredman B, White PF. Recovery following outpatient anesthesia: use of enflurane versus propofol. *J Clin Anesth* 1993;**5**:447–50.

18   Valanne J. Recovery and discharge of patients after long propofol infusion vs isoflurane anaesthesia for ambulatory surgery. *Acta Anaesthesiol Scand* 1992;**36**:530–3.

19   Smiley RM, Ornstein E, Matteo RS, Pantuck EJ, Pantuck CB. Desflurane and isoflurane in surgical patients: comparison of emergence times. *Anesthesiology* 1991;**74**:425–8.

20   Ghouri AF, Bodner M, White PF. Recovery profile after desflurane-nitrous oxide versus isoflurane-nitrous oxide in outpatients. *Anesthesiology* 1991;**74**:419–24.

21   Dexter F, Tinker JH. Comparisons between desflurane and isoflurane or propofol on time to following commands and time to discharge. A metaanalysis. *Anesthesiology* 1995;**83**:77–82.

22   Song D, Joshi GP, White PF. Fast-track eligibility after ambulatory anesthesia: a comparison of desflurane, sevoflurane, and propofol. *Anesth Analg* 1998;**86**:267–73.

23   Hough MB, Sweeney B. Postoperative nausea and vomiting in arthroscopic day-case surgery: a comparison between desflurane and isoflurane. *Anaesthesia* 1998;**53**:910–4.

24   Philip BK, Kallar SK, Bogetz MS, Scheller MS, Wetchler BV, Sevoflurane Multicenter Ambulatory Group. A multicenter comparison of maintenance and recovery with sevoflurane or isoflurane for adult ambulatory anesthesia. *Anesth Analg* 1996;**83**:314–19.

25   Tarazi EM, Philip BK. A comparison of recovery after sevoflurane or desflurane in ambulatory anesthesia. *J Clin Anesth* 1998;**10**:272–7.

26 Nathanson MH, Fredman B, Smith I, White PF. Sevoflurane versus desflurane for outpatient anesthesia: a comparison of maintenance and recovery profiles. *Anesth Analg* 1995;**81**:1186–90.

27 Van Hemelrijck J, Smith I, White PF. Use of desflurane for outpatient anesthesia: a comparison with propofol and nitrous oxide. *Anesthesiology* 1991;**75**:197–203.

28 Smith I, Ding Y, White PF. Comparison of induction, maintenance and recovery characteristics of sevoflurane-N$_2$O and propofol-sevoflurane-N$_2$O with propofol-isoflurane-N$_2$O. *Anesth Analg* 1992;**74**:253–9.

29 Philip BK, Lombard LL, Philip JH. Vital capacity induction with sevoflurane in adult surgical patients (letter). *J Clin Anesth* 1996;**8**:426.

30 Baker CE, Smith I. Sevoflurane: a comparison between vital capacity and tidal breathing techniques for the induction of anaesthesia and laryngeal mask airway placement. *Anaesthesia* 1999;**54**:841–4.

31 Yurino M, Kimura H. Induction of anesthesia with sevoflurane, nitrous oxide, and oxygen: a comparison of spontaneous ventilation and vital capacity rapid inhalation induction (VCRII) techniques. *Anesth Analg* 1993;**76**:598–601.

32 Hamilton JG. Needle phobia: a neglected diagnosis. *J Fam Pract* 1995;**41**:169–75.

33 Smith I, Johnson IT. Inhalation induction with sevoflurane reduces maintenance anesthetic costs (abstract). *Anesthesiology* 1998;**89**:A39.

34 Dashfield AK, Birt DJ, Thurlow J, Kestin IG, Langton JA. Recovery characteristics using single-breath 8% sevoflurane or propofol for induction of anaesthesia in day-case arthroscopy patients. *Anaesthesia* 1998;**53**:1062–6.

35 Thwaites AJ, Smith I. A double blind comparison of sevoflurane *versus* propofol and mivacurium for tracheal intubation in day case wisdom tooth extraction (abstract). *Br J Anaesth* 1998;**80**:A36.

36 Thwaites AJ, Edmends S, Tomlinson AA, Kendall JB, Smith I. A double-blind comparison of sevoflurane *vs* propofol and succinylcholine for tracheal intubation in children. *Br J Anaesth* 1999;**83**:410–14.

37 Hall JE, Henderson KA, Oldham TA, Pugh S, Harmer M. Environmental monitoring during gaseous induction with sevoflurane. *Br J Anaesth* 1997;**79**:342–5.

38 Smith I. Costs of sevoflurane and propofol anaesthesia–in reply (letter). *Br J Anaesth* 2000;**84**:418.

39 Logan M. Breathing systems: effect of fresh gas flow rate on enflurane consumption. *Br J Anaesth* 1994;**73**:775–8.

40 Nel MR, Ooi R, Lee DJH, Soni N. New agents, the circle system and short procedures. *Anaesthesia* 1997;**52**:364–7.

41 Mapleson WW. The theoretical fresh-gas flow sequence at the start of low-flow anaesthesia. *Anaesthesia* 1998;**53**:264–72.

42 Calvey TN, Williams NE. *Principles and practice of pharmacology for anaesthetists*, 3rd edn. Oxford: Blackwell, 1997.

43 Tramèr M, Moore A, McQuay H. Omitting nitrous oxide in general anaesthesia: meta-analysis of intraoperative awareness and postoperative emesis in randomized controlled trials. *Br J Anaesth* 1996;**76**:186–93.

44 Shakir AAK, Ramachandra V, Hasan MA. Day surgery postoperative nausea and vomiting at home related to peroperative fentanyl. *J One-day Surg* 1997;**6**(3):10–11.

45 Sukhani R, Vazquez J, Pappas AL, Frey K, Aasen M, Slogoff S. Recovery after propofol with and without intraoperative fentanyl in patients undergoing ambulatory gynecologic laparoscopy. *Anesth Analg* 1996;**83**:975–81.

46 Rosenblum M, Weller RS, Conard PL, Falvey EA, Gross JB. Ibuprofen provides longer lasting analgesia than fentanyl after laparoscopic surgery. *Anesth Analg* 1991;**73**:255–9.

47 Munday IT, Ward PM, Sorooshian S *et al*. Interaction between remifentanil and isoflurane in spontaneously breathing patients during ambulatory surgery (abstract). *Anesthesiology* 1995;**83**:A23.

48 Song D, Joshi GP, White PF. Titration of volatile anesthetics using bispectral index facilitates recovery after ambulatory anesthesia. *Anesthesiology* 1997;**87**:842–8.

49 Thwaites AJ, Smith I. BIS during TCI propofol or sevoflurane anesthesia (abstract). *Anesthesiology* 1998;**89**:A899.

50 Einarsson S, Bengtsson A, Stenqvist O, Bengtson JP. Decreased respiratory depression during emergence from anesthesia with sevoflurane/N$_2$O than with sevoflurane alone. *Can J Anaesth* 1999;**46**:335–41.

51 Djaiani G, Ribes-Pastor MP. Propofol auto-co-induction as an alternative to midazolam co-induction for ambulatory surgery. *Anaesthesia* 1999;**54**:63–7.

52 Dingley J, Ivanova-Stoilova TM, Grundler S, Wall T. Xenon: recent developments. *Anaesthesia* 1999;**54**:335–46.

53 Goto T, Saito H, Shinkai M, Nakata Y, Ichinose F, Morita S. Xenon provides faster emergence from anesthesia than does nitrous oxide-sevoflurane or nitrous oxide-isoflurane. *Anesthesiology* 1997;**86**:1273–8.

4: Intravenous anaesthesia

John Peacock

Overview

In considering the use of the intravenous route for induction and maintenance of anaesthesia, the basic aims of anaesthesia are still the same, i.e. a technique which provides loss of consciousness with absence of awareness and adequate depth of anaesthesia to ensure control of physical and physiological responses. Since no patient and no surgical procedure are ever "standard" or static, a technique must also allow for adjustment of depth of anaesthesia according to the patient response and the surgical stimulus. Therefore, there can never be a single "recipe" which will always fulfil such requirements. Principles need to be applied which permit the above aims to be achieved.

As individuals have attempted to introduce intravenous anaesthesia into their practice, there have been occasions where a recipe, such as the step-down "Bristol regimen" for a manual infusion of propofol, has been quoted as the "dose to be used". The "10, 8, 6" (mg/kg/h) infusion scheme for propofol[1] was never intended to provide adequate anaesthesia for a fit young patient as the sole agent, with no adjustment for patient characteristics, surgical stimulus or concomitant anaesthetic agents. Such simplistic thinking has resulted in technical failure and a reluctance to use the technique further. As a consequence, the use of intravenous anaesthesia has not progressed as it could have with good education and appropriate selection of patients and techniques.

The aim of this chapter is to identify clear principles that can be applied to provide effective and safe intravenous anaesthesia in the day care setting whilst avoiding the extravagant and unsubstantiated claims of the enthusiast. The reality for the "generalist" is that there are potential advantages to be gained from the use of intravenous anaesthesia, but a single technique is not always applicable or superior and a degree of persistence is required to acquire familiarity with any technique before its advantages are reliably reproduced.

Aims of day case anaesthesia

In many respects the aims are the same as for any anaesthetic: a rapid smooth induction, stable adjustable anaesthesia, and rapid recovery. There should be minimal unwanted effects, as for any patient, but specifically for day case patients there is the concern to minimise the risk of postoperative nausea and vomiting (PONV) to ensure that discharge is not delayed. Any day case technique should also emphasise the need to provide good early postoperative analgesia (Chapter 7) which, with a clear-headed recovery, should permit early mobilisation and discharge. In combination with appropriate analgesic techniques, intravenous anaesthesia is at least as effective as any other form of anaesthesia in fulfilling these aims.

Recommendations for the selection of day case patients and procedures have focused on straightforward cases that have involved a shorter duration of anaesthesia and have usually required simpler forms of postoperative analgesia. This has meant that the anaesthetic technique has also been relatively uncomplicated. Increasingly procedures are more complex, of longer duration, require more sophisticated postoperative analgesia and involve patients who are less fit. The techniques we use in anaesthesia therefore need to continue to develop to reliably fulfil our aims of good control and rapid recovery.

Relative merits of intravenous anaesthesia

The major advantages and disadvantages of intravenous anaesthesia are listed in Box 4.1. The initial claim for intravenous anaesthesia was that the speed and quality of recovery was significantly superior to that from inhalational agents. With the advent of the newer short-acting agents sevoflurane and desflurane, the actual speed of recovery and time to achieve a clear-headed state is probably very little different. However, the main advantage of intravenous anaesthesia remains that propofol provides a much-improved recovery due to a significantly lower incidence of PONV, even compared to techniques using the newer inhalational agents.[2]

Box 4.1 The relative merits of intravenous anaesthesia

Positive	*Negative*
• Low incidence of PONV	• Increased cost of disposables
• Rapid increase in depth of anaesthesia	• Increased direct drug costs
• Drug delivery independent of ventilation	• No direct measure of drug concentration
• Some agents reversible	• Recovery dependent upon metabolism

PONV, postoperative nausea and vomiting

Another significant advantage of intravenous anaesthetic agents is that administration and uptake remain in the direct control of the anaesthetist whether the patient is breathing spontaneously or has ventilation controlled. During inhalational administration of anaesthetic agents, hypoventilation or apnoea reduce or prevent further administration of drug and this therefore results in the depth of anaesthesia becoming lighter or at least prevents anaesthesia being deepened rapidly. With intravenous administration, respiration has no effect on the administration or uptake of drug and adjustment of the depth of anaesthesia remains in the control of the anaesthetist and therefore continues during hypoventilation, apnoea or laryngospasm. Additional increments of drug can therefore be administered and the depth of anaesthesia deepened rapidly as the need arises, whether this is in anticipation of an increase in surgical stimulus or a response to events, such as movement, that have already demonstrated an inadequate depth of anaesthesia.

In contrast, excretion of intravenous agents is independent of any degree of control by the anaesthetist, whereas respiration may be modified to increase excretion of an inhalational agent. Although a degree of patience will usually result in recovery of consciousness in a reasonable time frame, a further advantage of intravenous anaesthesia is that, where required, opioids and benzodiazepines are reversible with specific antagonists. This is becoming less of a problem as newer drugs, such as remifentanil, are specifically developed with rapid elimination to ensure rapid and reliable recovery.

Clearly there is no single agent, intravenous or inhalational, which can provide an ideal balance between anaesthesia and analgesia. However, recognition of the need to provide varying depths of anaesthesia and analgesia independently indicates a need to administer intravenous analgesic agents, which will often be synergistic with the hypnotic agent. Even where an inhalation agent maintains hypnosis, administration of intravenous analgesia by infusion allows greater degrees of control over the depth of anaesthesia.

One of the potential disadvantages of intravenous anaesthesia is the apparent cost. Many have quoted the relative cost of the infusion pumps and the disposables associated with the use of the expensive intravenous agents and neglected the cost of the vaporiser in their comparison. In terms of the simple cost of the agents, the intravenous techniques are more expensive. However, when the cost of the increased use of antiemetics and possible delay in discharge with increased nursing time and admission rates are taken into consideration and set against the cost of the surgical procedure and theatre time, the cost of the intravenous technique has minimal effect.[3] This is especially so if the quality of recovery and discharge is superior.

Choice of anaesthetic agents and technique

Induction

Until recently, there was no expectation that anything other than the intravenous route would be used to induce anaesthesia in the fit adult day case patient, although the occasional exception might be permitted for a patient with a severe needle phobia. With the development of sevoflurane in particular, there is now the possibility that an inhalational agent can be seriously considered for induction of anaesthesia.[4] However, rapid loss of consciousness does not necessarily indicate adequate depth of anaesthesia for surgery to commence.

There is a wide choice of agents for intravenous induction of anaesthesia and theoretically, almost any agent could be used. The majority of agents were developed to use as a single dose, followed by another agent for maintenance. Under these conditions, differences in later recovery or hospital discharge may not always be apparent depending upon what agent is used for maintenance. However, the differences between the induction agents has become more important as speed of initial recovery and return of psychomotor skills has improved with the newer maintenance agents, be they inhalational or intravenous.

Etomidate and methohexital (methohexitone) have both been suggested as appropriate selections for day case induction at some stage. Unwanted side effects, such as movement and pain on injection, have limited their use, however. Similar effects are also seen with propofol but these seem to have been overcome with the use of lidocaine (lignocaine), administered prior to induction or mixed with the propofol, and the use of concomitant agents. Propofol has become the agent of choice,[5] primarily due to a rapid smooth induction and the ability to insert an airway earlier than with other agents. It is also due to the reduced incidence of PONV following propofol and to the rapid return of psychomotor function compared to thiopental (thiopentone) where psychomotor skills may still be impaired 24 hours after administration. The fact that propofol is also the IV agent most frequently used as the hypnotic for maintenance simplifies the anaesthetic technique, although the "single agent for induction and maintenance" has also been proposed for sevoflurane.[6] The use of ketamine has been proposed due to its analgesic effects although it has variable onset time, a longer recovery period, and particular problems with dreams and hallucinations.

Maintenance

The choice of intravenous agent for maintenance of day case anaesthesia is primarily directed towards those that are rapidly metabolised and result in rapid and clear-headed recovery. Although longer acting agents such as thiopental can theoretically be infused to adequately maintain anaesthesia, recovery is inevitably delayed, which makes it completely unsuitable for day case surgery. As indicated above, any intravenous agent which is rapidly metabolised (e.g. methohexital) could be used to maintain anaesthesia but etomidate and other agents have proven unsuitable due to unwanted side effects. Propofol, in practical terms, is the agent that is used with most frequency due to its pharmacokinetic advantages and the low incidence of PONV associated with its use.

Administration of intravenous anaesthetics

In order to maintain anaesthesia with intravenous agents, the drug needs to be administered to take account of early redistribution, intermediate transfer of drug within the body and elimination from the body–the BET (bolus, elimination, and transfer) scheme. Since short-acting drugs which are rapidly excreted are ideal for day case recovery, a system with an initial loading dose (bolus) and an infusion that can be adjusted to take account of both transfer and elimination is most useful, rather than repeat administration of increments. Manual infusion schemes can be based on an infusion supplemented by increments as clinically indicated or a step-down infusion such as the "Bristol scheme".[1] Although infusions that are adjusted manually are possible, the development of computer-controlled infusions, which automatically alter the infusion rate exponentially to adjust for redistribution and elimination, has made the practicality of intravenous anaesthesia much easier for the majority of anaesthetists.[7] Propofol has the added advantage that it can be administered by a licensed target-controlled infusion (TCI) system.

This does not preclude the use of manual infusion schemes, especially for agents that have a very short half-life and therefore equilibrate very rapidly. Remifentanil, which will be discussed in greater detail later, is such an agent and has an almost linear relationship between the infusion rate and the blood concentration after a relatively short period of infusion. This means that a change in infusion rate will be reflected within 5–10 minutes by a proportional change in the blood concentration and this will negate some of the advantages of TCI.

Target-controlled infusions

The advent of TCI has provided a significant degree of confidence to many using intravenous anaesthesia. There appears to be a greater degree of assurance in using the target in a similar way to the end-tidal concentration or the percentage set on the vaporiser. However, it is important to recognise that population pharmacokinetics are used in the computer calculations to adjust the infusion rate to produce a theoretical blood concentration at any given time, just as the minimum alveolar concentration (MAC) is defined as a response in 50% of individuals. Thus, between individuals, there will be variable accuracy in the actual blood concentration achieved, as each patient will handle the drug differently.[8] This pharmacokinetic variability should not hinder the use of TCI, since the administration of all anaesthetic drugs should be adjusted according to the individual patient response.

There is also additional variability between individuals in the sensitivity of the patient to any given blood concentration and this pharmacodynamic variability will change as the target concentration is adjusted to take account of differences in surgical stimulus. Therefore just, as there is no single end- tidal concentration of an inhalation agent which will always provide perfect anaesthesia, so there is no single target concentration of intravenous agent that can be used to provide ideal anaesthetic conditions in all circumstances.

Concomitant agents

Having identified that propofol *via* a TCI is the method of choice for maintenance of hypnosis, there remains the question of whether it should be used as a single agent or in combination with other agents. Since the majority of day case patients do not need, or necessarily have time for, premedication before induction, the use of propofol as a sole agent requires the administration of much higher doses to ensure adequate anaesthesia than many anaesthetists are used to. This problem has already been mentioned with reference to the use of the Bristol regimen.[1]

The options available for the concomitant agent are varied and include inhalational and intravenous components. Nitrous oxide may increase the incidence of PONV but will reduce the dose of propofol whilst providing additional analgesia and reduce the incidence of awareness. Alternatively a benzodiazepine, such as midazolam, may be used as co-induction to reduce the initial requirement of propofol and speed induction. However, it provides no analgesic component and its relatively short duration of effect may not significantly reduce the maintenance dose of propofol. Ketamine in low dose has analgesic properties but the concerns regarding emergence phenomena remain.

The most common method utilised is to administer an opioid. This may be a small increment of fentanyl or alfentanil as co-induction, which will also provide analgesia that may last into the early postoperative recovery phase. Small increments of morphine or pethidine (meperidine), *via* the intravenous or intramuscular route, will reduce the dose requirement for propofol, may also be useful for postoperative analgesia and will not significantly depress respiration for prolonged periods. Unfortunately, the routine intraoperative administration of the longer acting opioids may significantly increase the incidence of PONV, reduce the speed of recovery and even increase the number of patients requiring admission. A more recent addition to the available choices for an opioid as part of the maintenance of anaesthesia is an infusion of remifentanil.

Remifentanil was specifically developed for very rapid elimination when used as an intravenous agent by infusion, so as to permit titration according to response and rapid recovery. This fast elimination is due to its metabolism by non-specific esterases in the blood and tissues. This results in an elimination half-life of 8–15 minutes and means that recovery following its use is extremely rapid. Recovery from remifentanil is virtually independent of infusion duration, age, hepatic or renal function and genetic disposition.[9] Since, in common with the other opioids, remifentanil is synergistic for its anaesthetic effects with propofol, the dose of propofol required to maintain an adequate depth of anaesthesia is significantly reduced.

Recovery

Recovery from anaesthesia is clearly affected by a number of factors, as discussed above, but will primarily be dependent upon the drug(s) selected and the dose(s) administered. Perhaps the ideal pharmacokinetic profile for an agent for day case anaesthesia would be a drug with rapid onset, rapid distribution, and extensive metabolism. Many of the current drugs fulfil the first two criteria but fail in the extent to which they are rapidly and extensively metabolised. Following distribution of considerable quantities of drug to the peripheral tissues over a period of 1–2 hours, this reservoir of drug returns to the circulation and acts to delay recovery. Alfentanil is initially short acting due to distribution to peripheral tissues, but has a slow recovery following prolonged infusion, due to redistribution from the peripheral reservoir back into the circulation prior to metabolism.

The term "context-sensitive half-time" was developed[10] to explain the fact that, for the majority of intravenous agents, the recovery time varies with, and is dependent upon, the duration of the infusion, even though the pharmacokinetics (e.g. distribution and elimination half-life, clearance) of the agent do not change during its administration. Context-sensitive half-time is defined as the time taken for a 50% reduction in the concentration of the drug and is therefore an indication of the rate of clinical recovery. Although propofol has extensive metabolism and is recognised as having rapid recovery, the context-sensitive half-time increases from approximately 10 minutes at one hour to 25 minutes at four hours. By comparison, remifentanil is metabolised so rapidly in the tissues, the blood, and liver that however long the infusion, there is no change in the context-sensitive half-time of approximately five minutes. That is not to say that the recovery time is always the same. The recovery *time* will be dependent upon the actual infusion rate of remifentanil used although the *rate* of recovery will be consistent, whatever dose is administered. A useful analogy is that it takes longer to climb down from the top of Everest than from the top of Ben Nevis although the rate of descent may be the same. This has not always been clearly explained and, whenever possible, the dose of remifentanil needs to be adjusted towards the end of surgery (just as with any other agent, be it inhalational or intravenous) to permit rapid recovery from a lower drug concentration.

However, the rate of recovery is not dependent upon the dose of a single drug but will be dependent upon the dose of all drugs used. Vuyk and colleagues[11] calculated the optimum target concentrations of alfentanil (and other opioids) with propofol to produce the ideal balance between adequate anaesthesia and rapid recovery. Increasing the concentration of propofol or alfentanil increased the recovery time, despite reducing the concentration of the other drug, since the drug with the higher concentration produced longer lasting effects. This balance of effects may be altered where the two drugs do not have similar rates of excretion. In this case, the greatest emphasis should be placed on the drug with the significantly greater excretion. Thus the emphasis of anaesthesia could realistically be placed on remifentanil, which will be excreted significantly faster than propofol, permitting a lower concentration of propofol to ensure loss of consciousness. Thus as remifentanil is rapidly metabolised the recovery from a lower dose of propofol will be significantly faster than that where higher concentrations of propofol were used to maintain adequate anaesthesia as previously calculated.[11] Care should be taken not to reduce the level of propofol too far, however, or awareness may be a risk.[12]

Opioid-based or opioid-supplemented anaesthesia

This concept can be extended since the introduction of remifentanil to present another addition to the choices regarding drug selection and dose administration. Previously, the selection of a particular opioid has been based upon the duration of intraoperative and postoperative effect, with the dose administered chosen to avoid respiratory depression or other side effects during recovery. As a result, the dose administered was often lower than optimal to prevent responses during surgery, in order to minimise the unwanted effects in the postoperative period. This is opioid-*supplemented* anaesthesia and it is effective in reducing the required dose of hypnotic drug but does not completely ablate responses to surgery.

However, since remifentanil is so rapidly metabolised and the rate of recovery is so rapid whatever the dose of remifentanil administered, there is now the option to change to opioid-*based* anaesthesia, with remifentanil being administered in significantly higher doses in order to prevent responses to surgery. The dose of hypnotic is then administered at a much lower rate of infusion, with the prime aim being to ensure lack of awareness rather than contribute significantly to the depth of anaesthesia. Recovery can still be fast, since anaesthesia has been based on a drug which will not be detectable in the circulation within an hour. Awareness should not be a problem provided that an adequate amount of hypnotic is still delivered. Nevertheless, remifentanil (and other opioids) may abolish many of the *signs* of awareness and vigilance is therefore essential.

Practicalities of intravenous anaesthesia

Induction

One of the perceived problems of a TCI system is that induction is much slower than the majority of people are used to and this may cause significant delay on a day case list. This occurs because the loading dose of propofol using a TCI is much smaller than the loading dose administered using a manual scheme. It therefore takes longer for the patient to reach an adequate depth of anaesthesia for an airway to be inserted or for surgery to commence.

When the Bristol scheme was first introduced, a loading dose of 1 mg/kg was used[1] and this was smaller than the 2–2.5 mg/kg that was currently being recommended. This was further exaggerated by investigations that were using infusions of propofol for induction of anaesthesia to try and identify the actual doses of propofol required for induction and how this varied with age.[13] This was prompted by concerns expressed following the introduction of propofol that it resulted in a much greater reduction in arterial pressure than the currently available drugs. Doses of 0.8–1.2 mg/kg were identified as being adequate to induce anaesthesia without significant reductions in arterial pressure but with obvious variations in individual response according to increasing age, ASA status, premedication, and concomitant administration of other drugs. At the same time, induction with a TCI system was shown not to result in significant reductions in arterial pressure at targets of 5 µg/ml.[14]

Since then, it has been recognised that the target concentration selected for induction will need to be adjusted according to the factors listed above. Having selected a particular target concentration for induction, the Diprifusor® calculates the loading dose and administers this at approximately 1200 ml/h, which is equivalent to 200 mg over one minute. A range of the loading doses that would be administered using the Diprifusor® for a selection of patient weights and initial target concentrations is shown in Table 4.1.

Table 4.1 Induction dose and administration time using different initial target concentrations. Values were generated by the Diprifusor® for a 40-year-old patient

Target concentration (µg/ml)	Loading dose and duration of administration Weight of patient		
	50 kg	*70 kg*	*90 kg*
4	4.6 ml, 13 s	6.4 ml, 19 s	8.2 ml, 24 s
6	6.9 ml, 20 s	9.6 ml, 28 s	12.3 ml, 37 s
8	9.1 ml, 27 s	12.8 ml, 38 s	16.5 ml, 49 s

Overpressure

In order to increase the speed of induction and reduce the time delay that can occur before the commencement of surgery, a technique similar to that of over-pressure in inhalational anaesthesia can be utilised. Instead of the target which would be used for initial maintenance of anaesthesia being selected for induction and the blood (and brain) concentration gradually reaching this value, a higher target is selected in order to increase the initial loading dose administered, as in Table 4.1. Even with a significant increase in the target concentration from 4 to 8 μg/ml, the loading dose for a 90 kg individual is increased from only 82 mg to 165 mg which is still significantly less than the 200 mg frequently administered as the induction dose by hand. Target concentrations of 4 and 8 μg/ml approximate to loading doses of 0.9 and 1.8 mg/kg.

When loss of consciousness is achieved, the target concentration is reduced in order to prevent the TCI delivering propofol in larger amounts to maintain this artificially high initial concentration. Leaving the selected target concentration at the higher value would result in greater depth of anaesthesia than required and the risk of unwanted effects such as hypotension. This selection of an initial high target followed by a rapid reduction to the required maintenance target will reduce the likelihood of unwanted effects associated with the higher dose but increase the speed of induction. This occurs because the higher initial plasma concentration provides a steeper gradient down which drug can flow into the site of drug action (the "effect site"). Reducing the plasma concentration shortly before the desired effect site concentration is achieved causes the effect site to equilibrate at the desired level much earlier than if this value is entered as the initial plasma target (Fig. 4.1). This will enable earlier management of the airway, if appropriate, or surgery to commence sooner than if the lower target was selected from the outset. Early equilibration between plasma and effect site ensures that subsequent changes in plasma concentration are rapidly reflected at the effect site.

Ventilation

As part of the initial anaesthesia plan, the decision has to be made on how the airway will be managed. The options have been discussed in Chapter 2 but this choice will influence how the anaesthetic drugs are selected and administered. Will a simple facemask be used, a laryngeal mask inserted or will the patient's trachea be intubated? Will the aim be to use spontaneous or assisted ventilation? There will be some specific indications, be they surgical or anaesthetic, where intubation is preferred and others where assisted ventilation is appropriate; however, there are many day case scenarios where insertion of a laryngeal mask and spontaneous ventilation would appear to be the most effective technique.

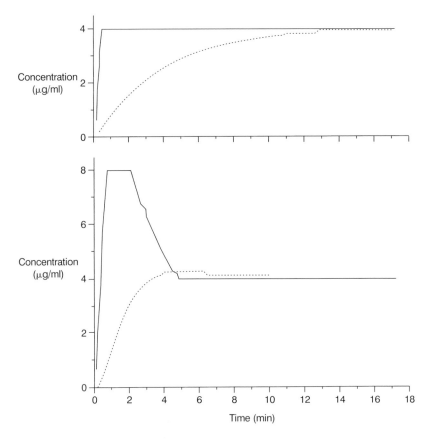

Figure 4.1 *Upper panel*: A target-controlled infusion (TCI) system set to deliver a plasma concentration of 4 μg/ml rapidly achieves and maintains this value (solid line). The concentration in the effect site (dashed line) rises much more slowly, however, and does not reach equilibration with plasma until nearly 18 minutes.
Lower panel: Using "overpressure" the plasma target (solid line) is initially set at 8 μg/ml, but reduced to 4 μg/ml after insertion of a laryngeal mask airway. The effect site concentration (dashed line) reaches the desired value of 4 μg/ml within four minutes and is subsequently maintained at about this level with only a slight overshoot. Data for the overpressure regimen were derived from clinical experiment;[2] all concentrations were simulated using the Diprifusor®.

Where a laryngeal mask is to be inserted, adequate depth of anaesthesia is required which is then frequently followed by a period of apnoea, especially if an opioid has been used in the induction sequence. This could be considered by some as undesirable or a failure of technique. However, as anaesthetists, we are trained to manage the airway and the requirement to squeeze a bag by hand or *via* a ventilator as part of a circle system would not in general be detrimental to the patient.

The next decision is whether to try and achieve spontaneous ventilation as soon as possible or maintain deep anaesthesia and leave recovery of respiration until the end of surgery. Within the context of superficial surgery using a laryngeal mask, the obvious preference is to try and achieve spontaneous ventilation during the procedure. This will permit the patient to be transferred to recovery as soon as surgery is finished, rather than leave it to the end of surgery where continued apnoea will inevitably delay the start of the next patient and slow the progress of the operating list.

Use of spontaneous ventilation also offers the opportunity to gain confidence in the use of techniques and doses of drugs that prevent response to surgery and ensure loss of consciousness. When techniques are then transposed to intubated patients who have received neuromuscular blocking agents, there is a far greater confidence in the doses required to ensure lack of awareness.

Anaesthetic drug doses

In identifying the appropriate doses of intravenous agents to use, it is important to identify the actual combination of drugs being used and the order of their administration.

Table 4.2 Propofol infusion rates and whole blood concentrations with concomitant agents of lorazepam, morphine or temazepam premedication and nitrous oxide or alfentanil for maintenance. Data from references [16-18]

	Lorazepam / N_2O	Morphine / N_2O	Temazepam / alfentanil
ED_{95} (mg/kg/h)	20.9 (14.0–77.8)	6.7 (5.1–18.4)	5.0 (4.1–8.8)
EC_{95} (μg/ml)	5.9 (NA)	3.4 (NA)	4.1 (2.8–30.5)
ED_{50} (mg/kg/h)	7.8 (6.4–10.0)	3.2 (2.4–3.8)	2.9 (2.4–3.4)
EC_{50} (μg/ml)	2.5 (NA)	1.7 (NA)	1.4 (0.6–1.9)

$ED_{95/50}$ is the final infusion rate for 95% and 50% confidence, respectively, of no response to surgical stimulus (95% confidence limits). $EC_{95/50}$ is the whole blood concentration for 95 and 50% confidence, respectively, of no response. (NA = not available.)

The Bristol team published data on the effect of different premedication regimes on the dose requirements for propofol (Table 4.2). The effective dose, which in this case is a maintenance propofol infusion rate, which would prevent movement at incision in 95% of the population (ED_{95}) with lorazepam premedication and nitrous oxide supplementation was 20.9 mg/kg/h. This was with a range for the 95% confidence interval of 14.0 to 77.8 mg/kg/h. The effective plasma concentration in 95% of the population (EC_{95}), which would equate with the target concentration, was 5.9 μg/ml. Significant dose reductions were obtained by the use of an opioid, morphine

0.15 mg/kg as premedication or alfentanil during maintenance (see Table 4.2). Much lower doses of propofol are required to prevent movement as a response to surgery in the presence of neuromuscular blocking drugs. Scheepstra and colleagues[15] quoted effective maintenance infusion rates of 10 mg/kg/h in young people but in the presence of vecuronium and doses of fentanyl of 0.75–1.5 µg/kg every 30 minutes. It very quickly becomes apparent that the decision to select a given target concentration of propofol will depend upon what other drugs are simultaneously being administered.

The order of drug administration is important for the dose of each drug used and the side effect profile which may result. Induction commencing with propofol will require administration of high doses that may result in movement and may be followed by hypotension as it is supplemented by additional drugs. Commencing anaesthesia with an opioid before starting the propofol infusion will reduce the incidence of movement but increase the duration of apnoea following induction. At the present time there is no technique published where anaesthesia can be reliably induced and both movement and apnoea avoided in all cases, although careful titration of dose to response of the patient will achieve such conditions during surgery.

Suggested techniques

Two variations in technique that I have used with good effect are based upon the use of spontaneous ventilation with a laryngeal mask for superficial general surgery and assisted ventilation with an endotracheal tube for ophthalmic surgery. Either example would need to be modified to suit other circumstances but both demonstrate the principles described above. Both involve the use of propofol and remifentanil and preferentially avoid the use of nitrous oxide. Postoperative analgesia is principally provided by a combination of local anaesthesia and non-steroidal analgesics with the addition of longer acting opioids postoperatively where the above have failed. These techniques are described in detail below and are also summarised in Box 4.2.

Assisted ventilation with endotracheal tube

For fit healthy individuals who have not received other drugs as premedication, the following regime would be followed and adjusted according to individual response. In order to reduce the dose of propofol required for the induction of anaesthesia, the remifentanil infusion is commenced first. Since loading doses of remifentanil have been identified as resulting in muscular rigidity and apnoea, the loading dose is always administered as an infusion over 60 seconds, with the patient being warned that they may become light-headed. Since assisted ventilation is electively being used, the loading dose of remifentanil is the recommended 1 µg/kg/min. After this,

Box 4.2 Summary of practical propofol-remifentanil regimens for use during controlled and spontaneous ventilation (see text for more details)

Assisted ventilation with endotracheal tube

Induction	• Remifentanil 1 μg/kg/min for 1 min • Reduce remifentanil to 0.5 μg/kg/min • Start propofol at target of 8 μg/ml
At loss of consciousness	• Atracurium 0.15–0.25 mg/kg • Reduce propofol target to 4 μg/ml
Maintenance	• Remifentanil 0.2–0.5 μg/kg/min • Propofol 2–4 μg/ml • Aim for lower values towards end of case

Spontaneous ventilation with laryngeal mask

Induction	• Remifentanil 0.2 μg/kg/min for 30–60 s • Reduce remifentanil to 0.1 μg/kg/min • Start propofol at target of 8 μg/ml
At loss of consciousness	• Reduce propofol target to 4 μg/ml • Insert laryngeal mask and assist ventilation as needed
Maintenance	• Remifentanil 0.05–0.2 μg/kg/min • Propofol 2–4 μg/ml

---

the remifentanil infusion is reduced to 0.5 μg/kg/min, and the propofol infusion commenced at a target concentration of 8 μg/ml.

As soon as consciousness is lost, a small dose of atracurium (approximately 0.15–0.25 mg/kg) is given to prevent any cough on intubation and the target concentration of propofol is reduced to 4 μg/ml. At this stage, the estimated blood propofol concentration will not always have reached its target but the infusion rate will then be set to zero until the estimated blood concentration falls back to 4 μg/ml, at which point it recommences at the appropriate rate. Ventilation is assisted by hand to permit the atracurium to take effect before intubation takes place, primarily under the effects of the remifentanil and propofol. Muscular rigidity is rarely of sufficient severity to impede ventilation, although changes in chest wall compliance may be noticed as the atracurium takes effect. The use of infusions for both drugs rarely results in significant hypotension in fit patients.

The maintenance infusions of the two drugs are adjusted according to the response of the patient to surgery, with commonly used doses of 0.2–0.5 μg/kg/min for remifentanil and 2–4 μg/ml for propofol with ventilation using oxygen in air. Further doses of atracurium are not usually required, unless muscle relaxation is a particular surgical requirement, and reversal is rarely needed at the end of surgery. As experience is gained, the infusion rates of both hypnotic and opioid are reduced towards the very end of surgery so that the final infusion rates are in the region of 0.05 µg/kg/min for remifentanil and 2 µg/ml for propofol. When the infusion lines are flushed, this will provide a small additional dose but recovery of respiration and consciousness will occur rapidly within a few minutes. Since remifentanil provides no postoperative analgesia, the local anaesthesia and non-steroidal analgesics are preferentially administered at the beginning of surgery.

Spontaneous ventilation with laryngeal mask

In order to reduce the induction dose of propofol, the remifentanil infusion is again commenced first, but at a lower dose to expedite spontaneous respiration. Remifentanil is commenced at 0.2 µg/kg/min for 30–60 seconds and then continued at 0.1 µg/kg/min. The loading dose of remifentanil is therefore reduced by 5–10-fold. Again the propofol target concentration is selected to 8 µg/ml until loss of consciousness when it is reset to 4 µg/ml. As with the assisted ventilation scenario above, the target concentration may not have been reached, but the infusion rate will be set to zero until the estimated blood concentration reaches 4 µg/ml. Following loss of consciousness, apnoea will usually ensue but insertion of the laryngeal mask will easily be achieved within a short period of time. Where a circle anaesthesia system is available, respiration can easily be supported by moderately small tidal volumes at low respiratory rates to maintain an end tidal CO_2 in the region of 5–6 kPa. Alternatively the bag may be squeezed by hand.

Spontaneous respiration may restart after surgery has commenced or may require further dose reductions of either or both drugs, dependent upon patient variability. Remifentanil can be reduced in steps of 0.025–0.05 µg/kg/min or propofol by reducing the set target by 1 µg/ml increments. The maintenance doses of propofol and remifentanil will most frequently be in the range of 2–4 µg/ml and 0.05–0.2 µg/kg/min, respectively. These low infusion rates can be maintained until the end of surgery, when the infusions can be discontinued and the patient immediately transferred to the postanaesthetic recovery area where they will awake in a very short period of time.

Both of the above infusion regimens are based upon patients being fit and healthy. Significant dose reductions are recommended for both propofol and remifentanil in elderly patients to avoid side effects. The duration of apnoea and the degree of hypotension will be significantly increased if the above infusion rates are not reduced. Remifentanil has a recommended dose reduction of 50%, such that the loading dose over 60 seconds should be 0.5 µg/kg/min, or even lower in the presence of significant concomitant disease. Although the final maintenance target concentrations of propofol may be similar to those in younger patients, the initial loading dose should again be reduced and, dependent upon the degree of concomitant disease, may be as low as 4 μg/ml.

Summary

Induction of anaesthesia with intravenous anaesthetics is commonplace. Using the same intravenous drug for maintenance of anaesthesia offers control over the delivery of anaesthesia, independent of the ventilatory state of the patient. Using propofol as the hypnotic component of anaesthesia offers the additional advantages of rapid and smooth recovery with a low incidence of PONV.

Propofol alone is inadequate for anaesthesia (unless very large doses are administered) and requires analgesic supplementation with nitrous oxide and/or opioid analgesics. A short-acting opioid is desirable to facilitate rapid recovery and to reduce opioid side effects. Alfentanil has been popular in the past but remifentanil may be preferable because its extremely brief duration allows excellent intraoperative control and postoperative recovery.

Induction of anaesthesia with either of the infusion schemes described in detail will be rapid and controlled and yet will permit surgery to commence promptly. Unwanted movement resulting from the use of propofol is unusual due to the addition of remifentanil, which helps provide adequate depth of anaesthesia but inevitably results in apnoea in the early stages following induction. Recovery from the above infusion schemes will be rapid and reproducible, with patients having a low incidence of PONV. Where appropriate analgesia has been provided in a timely manner, postoperative pain should not be the significant problem previously reported following the use of remifentanil for major surgery. In addition, patients will be clear-headed and will therefore be eligible for early discharge from hospital. Clearly other techniques are also suitable for day case surgery but intravenous anaesthesia should be a technique that we are all sufficiently familiar with to use when other techniques are inappropriate.

1   Roberts FL, Dixon J, Lewis GTR, Tackley RM, Prys–Roberts C. Induction and mainte-nance of propofol anaesthesia. A manual infusion scheme. *Anaesthesia* 1988;**43**(suppl):14–17.
2   Smith I, Thwaites AJ. Target-controlled propofol *vs.* sevoflurane: a double-blind, randomised comparison in day-case anaesthesia. *Anaesthesia* 1999;**54**:745–52.
3   Rowe WL. Economics and anaesthesia. *Anaesthesia* 1998;**53**:782–8.
4   Thwaites A, Edmends S, Smith I. Inhalation induction with sevoflurane–a double-blind comparison with propofol. *Br J Anaesth* 1997;**78**:356–61.
5   Smith I, White PF, Nathanson M, Gouldson R. Propofol: an update on its clinical use. *Anesthesiology* 1994;**81**:1005–43.
6   Smith I, Thwaites AJ. VIMA and recovery with sevoflurane. *Acta Anaesthesiol Scand* 1998;**42**(suppl 112):219–21.

7   Glen JB. The development of 'Diprifusor': a TCI system for propofol. *Anaesthesia* 1998;**53**(suppl 1):13–21.

8   Swinhoe CF, Peacock JE, Glen JB, Reilly CS. Evaluation of the predictive performance of a 'Diprifusor' TCI system. *Anaesthesia* 1998;**53**(suppl 1):61–7.

9   Thompson JP, Rowbotham DJ. Remifentanil–an opioid for the 21st century (editorial). *Br J Anaesth* 1996;**76**:341–3.

10   Hughes MA, Glass PSA, Jacobs JR. Context-sensitive half-time in multicompartment pharmacokinetic models for intravenous anesthetic drugs. *Anesthesiology* 1992;**76**:334–41.

11   Vuyk J, Mertens MJ, Olofsen E, Burm AGL, Bovill JG. Propofol anesthesia and rational opioid selection. *Anesthesiology* 1997;**87**:1549–62.

12   Ogilvy AJ. Awareness during total intravenous anaesthesia with propofol and remifentanil (letter). *Anaesthesia* 1998;**53**:308.

13   Peacock JE, Spiers SPW, McLauchlan GA, Edmondson WC, Berthoud MC, Reilly CS. Infusion of propofol to identify effective doses for induction of anaesthesia in young and elderly patients. *Br J Anaesth* 1992;**69**:363–7.

14   Chaudhri S, White M, Kenny GNC. Induction of anaesthesia with propofol using a target-controlled infusion system. *Anaesthesia* 1992;**47**:551–3.

15   Scheepstra GL, Booij LHDJ, Rutten CLG, Coenen LGJ. Propofol for induction and maintenance of anaesthesia: comparison between younger and older patients. *Br J Anaesth* 1989;**62**:54–60.

16   Richards MJ, Skues MA, Jarvis AP, Prys-Roberts C. Total IV anaesthesia with propofol and alfentanil: dose requirements for propofol and the effect of premedication with clonidine. *Br J Anaesth* 1990;**65**:157–63.

17   Spelina KR, Coates DP, Monk CR, Prys-Roberts C, Norley I, Turtle MJ. Dose requirements of propofol by infusion during nitrous oxide anaesthesia in man. I: Patients premedicated with morphine sulphate. *Br J Anaesth* 1986;**58**:1080–4.

18   Turtle MJ, Cullen P, Prys-Roberts C, Coates D, Monk CR, Faroqui MH. Dose requirements of propofol by infusion during nitrous oxide anaesthesia in man. II: Patients premedicated with lorazepam. *Br J Anaesth* 1987;**59**:283–7.

5: Regional anaesthesia

JOHAN RÆDER

Overview

Regional anaesthesia offers the distinct benefits that only the operative site (or its immediate surroundings) needs to be anaesthetised. All the considerable disadvantages and hazards of general anaesthesia are thereby avoided. In addition, providing complete intraoperative pain relief ensures that analgesia will also be effective in the immediate postoperative period. Despite these apparent advantages, the use of regional anaesthesia for ambulatory surgery is highly variable from country to country and from region to region.

Ambulatory surgery is characterised by surgery of low or intermediate duration and invasiveness, stable, elective patients and high patient turnover. The principles of regional anaesthesia, its benefits and drawbacks, as well as proper selection and performance of techniques, will be discussed in this context.

Principles of regional anaesthesia

Regional anaesthesia implies using knowledge of the anatomy of the nervous system in order to anaesthetise a region of the body with a local anaesthetic agent. The regional techniques seek to identify specific nerves, or bundles of nerves, in order to block the impulses from the periphery into the central nervous system. This is in contrast to local anaesthesia, where diffuse infiltration of peripheral tissue blocks the pain at the nerve terminals in the surgical field. While theoretically superior, local anaesthesia is difficult to use for intermediate or major procedures, due to technical difficulties in blocking all structures involved and because of concern about the toxicity of high-dose local anaesthetic.

Thus, with regional anaesthesia, painful inputs are created in the surgical wound but they are blocked before, or as, they enter the spinal cord. In terms of pain physiology there are a lot of theoretical benefits to this approach. The pain-enforcing mechanisms in the spinal cord are not stimulated when an adequate regional block is applied and there is no wind-up or sensitisation. This differs from general anaesthesia, where noxious stimuli are allowed to enter and act in the central nervous system before they are

97

suppressed. Blocking pain before it is registered in the spinal cord is the basis of preemptive analgesia. This exciting concept has been proven in basic and animal research,[1] but is still controversial in clinical studies (see Chapter 7).

As the pain stimuli are blocked before entering the spinal cord, no systemic-acting drugs, with side effects such as nausea, somnolence or respiratory depression, are needed during surgery. As the block usually lasts for some time after the end of surgery, excellent pain relief is maintained during the first, most painful postsurgical phase.

Clinical benefits and drawbacks of regional anaesthesia

These may be discussed in terms of safety, quality, and economy and are summarised in Box 5.1.

Box 5.1 The relative merits of regional anaesthesia

Positive	*Negative*
• Effective intra- and postoperative analgesia	• Discomfort during block placement ± during procedure
• Avoids adverse effects of general anaesthetics:	• Delay in initiating some blocks
• low incidence of PONV	• Unacceptable to some patients/ surgeons/anaesthetists
• minimal postoperative somnolence	• Risk of nerve damage
• no respiratory depression	• Prolonged immobility/urinary retention with some blocks
• Patient may view operation and discuss findings	• Haemodynamic side effects with some blocks
• Patient more likely to bypass phase I recovery	• Technique may fail
• Reduced direct and indirect costs	

Safety

Properly performed ambulatory anaesthesia has a safety record of close to 100%, comparable with control groups of similar age not having surgery.[2] The study of Warner and colleagues also included a subgroup of patients having regional anaesthesia, but the number of patients (and major complications) in this and other studies are too low to say anything about the relative risks in terms of mortality or major complications.[2] However, some indication may be taken from studies of inpatients. In the American closed claims reports, regional anaesthesia fares favourably compared with general anaesthesia; the latter is more often associated with serious circulatory or respiratory complications, whereas regional anaesthesia has some reports of nerve injury.[3, 4] It is difficult to know the true incidence of such injuries, however, due to uncertainty as to the number of regional procedures performed. Spinal or epidural anaesthesia have been shown to improve regional blood flow and decrease the incidence of venous thrombosis in the lower extremities, although recent studies do not support the theory of differences in safety between regional or general anaesthesia when used in patients with cardiovascular or respiratory disease. However, as major adverse outcomes (or death) are very rare events, even in high-risk inpatients, almost all studies are underpowered in order to address these problems.

Recently, a large metaanalysis has been completed of 137 studies including 8292 patients with a random allocation to either regional anaesthesia (i.e. spinal or epidural) or general anaesthesia.[5] This metaanalysis showed significant benefits of the regional techniques in terms of reduced postoperative mortality, venous thromboses, pulmonary emboli, myocardial infarction, bleeding, pneumonia, respiratory depression, and renal failure.[5] Recent studies have also pointed out the risk of prolonged cognitive dysfunction in elderly patients after surgical procedures.[6] Whether or not regional anaesthesia is better in this respect is still controversial, although some studies in elderly orthopaedic inpatients provide evidence in favour of regional techniques.

Some major risks are specifically associated with regional anaesthetic techniques, however. An inadvertent intravenous injection or rapid absorption of a large dose of local anaesthetic may result in generalised convulsions and cardiac dysrhythmia or arrest. With epidural or spinal anaesthesia, the physiological changes associated with extended block of the sympathetic nervous system may result in hypotension, bradycardia or cardiac arrest. Supraclavicular or intercostal blocks may result in pneumothorax. Epinephrine (adrenaline) added to the distal local anaesthetic blocks, such as fingers, toes or penis, may result in ischaemia due to a poor collateral arterial blood supply. A prolonged postoperative spinal or epidural block will increase the risk of urinary retention, while a prolonged paralysed state in the lower body may increase the risk of pressure-induced nerve injury from the surroundings. Rare cases of spinal haematoma may more readily be overlooked if a prolonged paralysis is to be expected and a delay in the diagnosis of haematoma may increase the chances of permanent sequelae. With a prolonged stable block, there may be a further period of haemodynamic instability when the block wears off. The patient should be appropriately monitored and the anaesthetist should be prepared for treating this.

Quality

In terms of quality, less initial postoperative pain is an important feature with regional anaesthesia. There are also data to suggest that this initial pain relief also reduces the amount and severity of pain experienced after the block has worn off. In a study by Dahl and co-workers,[7] patients with epidural or spinal anesthesia had significantly less pain 1–2 hours after the block had worn off compared to the same period in patients who had received general anaesthesia. Both the absence of general anaesthetic after-effects and the reduced need for opioids for postoperative pain relief result in less postoperative nausea and vomiting when regional anaesthesia is used.[8]

With regional anaesthesia, patients have the option of choosing their perioperative conscious level. They may choose to stay fully awake, watching the TV screen of an arthroscope or discussing the operative findings with their surgeons. If patients specifically ask for this alternative, it is important not to use sedative drugs with a strong amnesic action, such as midazolam or propofol. Alternatives are music through headphones, chatting with the anaesthetist or nursing staff or receiving some sedation. The options for sedation are discussed more fully in Chapter 6.

Negative quality aspects of regional anaesthesia include pain during injection of local anaesthetics, occasional pain from the surgical site if the block is incomplete or deep structures are pulled on, and the problems associated with recovery from the block. The patient comfort of superior postoperative pain relief from, for example, a prolonged spinal block may be jeopardised by the anxiety some patients feel when their legs are totally paralysed for hours after the surgical procedure has finished. In some units, the intake of oral fluid and solids is restricted as long as the patients are paralysed, also adding to discomfort in the awake patient.

Economy

Whereas modern anaesthetic drugs for ambulatory general anaesthesia may be expensive to buy, the cost of drugs and equipment for regional anaesthesia is generally low.[8] The requirement for postoperative medication for pain or nausea relief may also be reduced with regional anesthesia, reducing indirect drug costs.

However, drug costs are only a minor part of the total costs associated with anaesthesia; most come from the use of labour and time in the highly dedicated operating theatre and recovery unit. A patient with regional anaesthesia may be wheeled directly out from the operating theatre after the surgeon has finished; no emergence, extubation or reestablishment of respiration and airway reflexes have to take place. Except for epidural and spinal anaesthesia, phase I recovery may often be bypassed (see Chapter 8), adding further to efficient postoperative care. A fully awake patient with no pain or nausea puts less workload on the recovery staff and, especially, the low rate of pain and nausea, is important in order to achieve a rapid discharge from phase I recovery or from the day case unit to home after ambulatory care.

The negative aspects of the cost of regional techniques may include extra preoperative time taken to establish a block and, for some blocks, to confirm that they are working properly. In the case of spinal or epidural anaesthesia, prolonged bed occupancy postoperatively, while waiting for the block to wear off, may also be a problem in terms of increased costs of nursing staff and reduced turnover in the day unit. If a patient is too heavily sedated during regional anaesthesia, sedation may persist into the postoperative period with reduced airway control, depressed respiration and delayed recovery, all adding to increased postoperative costs. Careful titration of sedation is clearly important and this is discussed in more detail in Chapter 6.

Minimising the dangers and drawbacks of regional anaesthesia

Consent from everybody involved

It is important for the success of regional anaesthesia to provide good information and establish consent for the technique, both from the surgeon and from the patient. If the patient is at all reluctant, every minor or major complaint in the perioperative period is likely to be attributed to the regional technique. In hospitals and patient populations not familiar with regional anaesthesia, surgeons may be puzzled and stressed by facing a patient who is awake. A regional anaesthetic technique sometimes calls for a more gentle surgical technique, while the options of prolonging the duration or extending the procedure may be limited. Furthermore, the conversation and attitudes in the operating room should take into consideration the fact that the patient may not be asleep. However, once regional anaesthesia becomes established as a successful department policy, previously reluctant surgeons and patients usually prefer this method as their first choice.[9]

Achieving optimal safety

Before the establishment of any regional technique, the patient should always have a standardised preanaesthetic interview and evaluation. An IV line and standard baseline monitoring (i.e. pulse oximetry, ECG, and regular BP readings) should be in place. Full preparation for any possible major complication should be undertaken, in terms of available equipment (suction, defibrillator, bag/mask, oxygen, intubation equipment), drugs (epinephrine, ephedrine, atropine, propofol or barbiturate, benzodiazepine, succinylcholine) and protocols for emergency action.

Drug toxicity
Epidural anaesthesia and brachial plexus block involve the delivery of local anaesthetics in high doses into highly vascularised tissue, which may result

101

in inadvertent intravascular injection or systemic absorption of neuro- or cardiotoxic doses of drug. Whereas generalised convulsions usually subside without sequelae, the cardiotoxic effect of high-dose bupivacaine is sometimes fatal. Therefore, when it is planned to use more than 10–15 ml of bupivacaine in an adult, the use of the less toxic ropivacaine or levobupivacaine should be encouraged.

Haemodynamic effects

With spinal or epidural anaesthesia, the subsequent extended sympathetic block may cause dangerous decreases in blood pressure and even bradycardia or cardiac arrest. Adequate hydration is therefore important and may also reduce postoperative nausea. This should not be overdone, however, as it may call for urinary catheterisation which, in general, should be avoided in ambulatory patients. A maximum of 500–1000 ml of electrolyte solution is recommended for a procedure with minimal blood loss; half of this volume should be given before or during neuraxial block administration. The patient should be observed closely and the anaesthetist should be prepared to give vasoconstrictors (e.g. ephedrine 5–10 mg IV) or atropine (0.5 mg IV) while symptoms of sympathetic block are evolving.

Spinal haematoma

Other feared complications of spinal or epidural anaesthesia are secondary infection and haematoma formation. Whereas postanaesthetic meningitis is extremely rare, a haematoma should always be considered if a block does not wear off within 4–5 hours after administration (or last supplement) or if the patient develops strong radiating pain some hours after placement of the block. Epidural or spinal blocks should be avoided in patients at high risk of haematoma formation, but may be used together with routine antithrombotic prophylaxis (used only in high-risk cases) and a maximum of one other antithrombotic agent (e.g. NSAID, dextran).[10]

In general, routine antithrombotic prophylaxis has not been advocated for ambulatory procedures with regional anaesthetic blocks, as the regional technique is sufficiently antithrombotic by itself compared with general anaesthesia. However, some units will advocate prophylaxis for prolonged operations when a tourniquet on the lower extremity is used.

Other complications

Intercostal or supraclavicular plexus blocks may cause pneumothorax, the onset of which is often delayed. For this reason, these blocks are not recommended for ambulatory patients. Permanent nerve damage may occur if a needle or an injection tears a nerve apart. However, this will create an intense radiating pain which is an important reason for having the patient awake and communicating while a regional block is performed. While a brief paraesthesia with a thin needle very rarely causes permanent harm, there is always the alternative of using nerve stimulators in order to avoid needle contact with the nerve. However, as the nerve-stimulating needles are usually thicker and more traumatic, they may also occasionally result in nerve damage.

The role of supplemental analgesia

Supplemental medication is considered more fully in Chapter 6. In terms of patient quality, all regional techniques involve the use of needles and are therefore associated with more or less pain. The perception of pain and preoperative anxiety may vary considerably between individual patients, as well as with different types of block and the skills of the anaesthetist. Whereas anxiolytic medication may be appropriate in some patients, too much may prevent patient cooperation during block placement while still not preventing the pain from the needle. A small dose of a rapidly acting opioid (e.g. alfentanil 0.5 mg in an adult) may be more appropriate for alleviation of unacceptable pain during painful block placement.

Bolus doses of alfentanil may also be appropriate if occasional pain occurs during the surgical procedure. If the perioperative pain is more frequent or long-lasting, a single bolus of fentanyl (50–150 μg) or an infusion of remifentanil (0.05–0.1 μg/kg/min) may be considered. However, when the pain is due to block failure, there should be a low threshold for (and minimal delay in) establishing either a new block or general anaesthesia. The latter may easily be accomplished by a bolus or infusion of propofol, with airway control established with a laryngeal mask airway. Anaesthesia may subsequently be supplemented with nitrous oxide and/or a volatile anaesthetic.

Time considerations

In terms of economy, the additional time required for placing the block and waiting for it to work before starting surgery may be a problem. In addition, there may be a delay in recovery of bladder function and haemodynamic stability after spinal or epidural anaesthesia. While spinal blocks and IV regional techniques may be established in the operating theatre without much delay compared with general anaesthesia, epidural and brachial plexus block may be better initiated in a preoperative holding area (or anaesthetic room), if one is available. If not, these blocks may be successfully applied in the operating theatre without much delay, provided that the scrub nurse is allowed to prepare and drape the patient while waiting for the block to become effective. The surgeon or the scrub nurse should then test the block in the operating field just before surgery starts. However, with such an approach, the anaesthetist should have some experience with the block and a clearcut strategy for rapid induction of general anaesthesia in the case of a block failure.

103

Suitability for regional anaesthesia

Suitable procedures

In general, all procedures which may be performed under regional anaesthesia in inpatients may also have regional blocks in the ambulatory setting. This includes all procedures in the extremities, including the shoulder, and all procedures beneath the umbilicus, including lower laparotomies. Superficial procedures on the trunk may also be performed with regional anaesthesia or local infiltration.

Some procedures are not suited for regional anaesthesia alone, such as upper laparotomies, major laparoscopies, and thoracotomies. There is no true regional technique for the head, face or neck although procedures in these regions may often be performed with local anaesthetic infiltration or single-nerve block. For procedures involving many regions simultaneously (e.g. skin grafting), regional techniques may not be appropriate due to the need for two concomitant blocks which may exceed the recommended maximum dose of local anaesthetic.

Suitable patients

All ambulatory surgical patients with a suitable procedure may have regional anaesthesia. In some cases, such as insulin-dependent diabetes or patients with symptoms of a mild upper airway infection, regional anaesthesia may be preferable to general anaesthesia. There are some exceptions, however.

• Patients who refuse a regional block in spite of proper information should not be forced to have a regional technique (see above), unless a strong contraindication to general anaesthesia is present.

• Patients with nerve injury or neurological deficit in the area of planned block should, in general, not have regional anaesthesia. Some exceptions may be appropriate, however, if general anaesthesia is strongly contraindicated or the patient has a strong preference for regional anaesthesia.

• Uncooperative patients are often poor subjects for regional anaesthesia. Again, the contraindication is relative and must be weighed against the alternatives. A useful approach is to induce hypnosis with a minimal amount of propofol or midazolam and then perform the block, leaving the patient able to react upon painful nerve stimulation or injection, before any permanent harm is done. In some children and elderly confused patients, such a combined approach of sleep and regional anaesthesia may be very successful.

• Infection at the site of the regional block is an absolute contraindication, such as an infected sacral cyst in the area of a planned caudal block.
• Anticoagulated patients should be evaluated even more strictly in the outpatient setting than as inpatients. A postoperative haematoma developing after discharge is even more dangerous in terms of ischaemia or nerve injury than it is in a more carefully observed inpatient (see above).

Choice of technique

Selection of blocks

The selection of blocks for an ambulatory anaesthetic practice should be adjusted according to the experience of the individual anaesthetist and how often he or she will have the opportunity of practising a specific block. The latter is a factor of both the case mix of the ambulatory unit and the frequency of attendance of the anaesthetist in question. As a minimum, every anaesthetist in ambulatory practice should master the spinal anaesthetic technique and have some sort of arm block (preferably a brachial plexus block technique) in their repertoire. The latter may be exchanged for an IV regional technique if their experience with brachial plexus blocks is very low. For regular practitioners of regional anaesthesia, a selection of other blocks may be added, the most useful ones in my experience being ankle block, interscalene (or parascalene) block, inguinal hernia block, femoral block, epidural block, and caudal block (in children). Depending on the case mix in the ambulatory unit, other blocks may also be useful, including paracervical block, eye blocks, sciatic nerve block, dorsal nerve of the penis block and specific blocks of nerves in the distal upper extremity, fingers, and toes.

Choice of local anaesthetic agent

For regional anaesthesia, a choice may have to be made of which drug to use, in which concentration and with which (if any) adjuvants. Local anaesthetic drugs may be divided into short acting (procaine, chloroprocaine), intermediate acting (lidocaine [lignocaine], prilocaine, mepivacaine) and long-acting (bupivacaine, levobupivacaine, and ropivacaine), dependent upon molecular characteristics.

Procaine and chloroprocaine are short acting because their ester structure renders them susceptible to degradation by pseudocholinesterase, an enzyme system which is widespread in the body fluids and, in most patients, has a high capacity for drug breakdown. However, ester degradation forms metabolites which may induce allergic reactions. The other local anaesthetic agents are all amides, which are predominantly degraded by liver enzymes. The capacity for degradation is therefore more limited but the risk of allergenic degradation products is far less than with the esters.

Whereas local anaesthetic infiltration should be accomplished with dilute preparations, more concentrated solutions are usually required in order to anaesthetise the thick nerves of a nerve bundle during a regional block. The addition of epinephrine in a 5–10 μg/ml concentration may be useful in order to speed up the onset, lower the toxicity and increase the duration of peripheral nerve blocks and epidural anaesthesia. With lidocaine, the addition of sodium bicarbonate, 0.5 mmol per 10 ml, may speed up the onset of some blocks. In addition, warm lidocaine may work faster than cold.

Lidocaine and bupivacaine are usually available in all parts of the world, whereas the availability of other local anaesthetic agents, such as mepivacaine, prilocaine, chloroprocaine, procaine, cocaine, ropivacaine, and levobupivacaine, may vary. In general, apart from using ropivacaine, or levobupivacaine for safety reasons for long-lasting high-dose blocks (see above), most anaesthetists will achieve their goals with only bupivacaine and lidocaine to hand. Lidocaine may be the drug of choice for spinal (see below) and epidural anaesthesia, for IV regional anaesthesia and for blocks for short-lasting procedures with little postoperative pain. Bupivacaine, with a slower onset and longer duration, may be the drug of choice for any prolonged cases and cases where prolonged postoperative analgesia is of high priority.

Spinal anaesthesia

Whereas drug doses for spinal anaesthesia are low and the risk of systemic toxicity may be negligible, the use of sharp needles and administration of concentrated drug into the spinal fluid involving direct contact with unprotected nerve tissue warrants utmost care. Spinal anaesthesia may result in some specific problems, such as the postdural puncture headache (PDPH), neurotoxic injury, and transient neurologic symptoms (TNS).

Choice of needle and the postdural puncture headache (PDPH)

In ambulatory surgery, the patients are usually mobilised with little or no surgical sequelae after discharge. In this setting, a PDPH lasting for days is unacceptable. The frequency of PDPH is related to age and to the size of the lesion in the dura when the spinal needle is withdrawn. PDPH has a rapidly declining incidence and severity in patients from 50 years of age and older, but may still be a serious problem in a very few elderly patients. The size of the dural lesion is related to the diameter of the needle and the needle design. The pencil-point design leaves a smaller puncture hole than an equally sized Quincke needle. Clinical studies also suggest that a smaller lesion, more valve-like, is produced by a Quincke needle when the puncture occurs *via* a lateral approach than with a midline approach. It is still disputed whether a Quincke bevel orientation parallel to the longitudinal dura fibres is better than other orientations. Whereas a 29 G Quincke needle carries a very low risk of PDPH, this very thin needle is hard to direct even with an introducer. Due to its narrow internal diameter, spinal fluid backflow is very slow and may add to the practical difficulties and extra time consumption when these needles are used. Furthermore, these extra-fine needles are more expensive than the pencil-point needles which, again, are somewhat more expensive compared with regular Quincke needles.

I use the 27 G pencil-point needle with an introducer as my routine spinal needle for all ambulatory cases. With a difficult back in an elderly patient, a 25 G or 22 G needle without introducer may sometimes be more easy to work with. If minor cost savings are an important issue, one may use a 25 or 27 G Quincke needle in patients above the age of 50 years.

With this approach, the incidence of mild PDPH should be in the 1–3% range, which should be acceptable as a minor postoperative problem. In some 0.5–1% of the spinal anaesthesia cases there will still be more severe headache, which may call for an epidural blood patch. It is therefore important to contact these patients the day after surgery for a standardised telephone follow-up, including questions of headache. Alternatively, the patients should have detailed information about this complication and the option of efficient blood patch therapy, if the symptoms are severe.

Toxicity and side effects

Whereas PHPH is related to needle size and design and not to drug characteristics, the opposite is the case for permanent nerve tissue damage (PNTD) and transient neurologic symptoms (TNS) (although nerve damage also may be caused by the needle trauma). Backache has been related to both the needle trauma and to chloroprocaine or, possibly, to the EDTA solvent in chloroprocaine.[11] PNTD and TNS are most frequently described with lidocaine, although both complications have also been reported after bupivacaine,[12] TNS after mepivacaine,[12] and PNTD after chloroprocaine.[13] Although lidocaine is involved with both TNS and PNTD, these seem to be two different issues, both pathophysiologically and clinically. TNS is benign, frequent, and self-limiting, without neurologic symptoms or sequelae. The frequency of TNS with spinal lidocaine varies considerably with study design: 0–5% if only spontaneous patient reports are considered, up to 20–40% when the patients are specifically asked about this symptom. The incidence is independent of lidocaine baricity, concentration or dose. TNS is more frequent in the lithotomy position or when the hip joint is frequently manipulated during anaesthesia, as with knee arthroscopy.[14] PNTD is rare but presents with neurologic symptoms and sometimes permanent paralysis. It is hardly ever described with less than

100 mg lidocaine in solutions of less than 50 mg/ml concentration.[15] With hyperbaric lidocaine, cases are also reported with doses less than 100 mg[15]. Whereas we do not know the pathophysiologic mechanism of TNS, neurotoxicity seems to be involved with PNTD. In fact, if we put an unprotected nerve in a lidocaine bath of more than 10–15 mg/ml concentration, this nerve will have permanent damage within 15–30 minutes.[16] Thus, when we use a concentrated lidocaine solution, we actually rely upon the dilution *in vivo* to be fast and efficient so as to avoid permanent damage. With high doses, slow injection, repeated injection or injection *via* a catheter this may not always be the case, so in these situations PNTD is more likely to occur.

Choice of drug

When a specific drug is chosen for spinal anaesthesia, the duration is also dose dependent. Thus, if the dose is low, even a long-acting drug may have a short clinical duration.[17] However, when the dose is reduced, there is an increased risk of inadequate block for surgery.[17] This risk may be reduced if an appropriate adjuvant drug, such as an opioid or an α_2 agonist, is used to lower the dose required.[18] Baricity may also influence the duration of action, by influencing the spread and dilution of drug in the spinal fluid. In a supine patient, a hyperbaric solution is distributed higher in the spinal fluid, resulting in some patients with a higher level of block with decreased intensity and decreased duration.[16] A rapid injection also tends to promote more widespread effect and shorter duration, whereas a slow injection through a side hole pencil-point needle spreads less, producing a denser, more localised, and longer lasting block.

Lidocaine
Lidocaine is the drug most frequently used for short-lasting spinal anaesthesia, due to a reliable effect lasting for 1–3 hours in a dose-dependent way. A minimum concentration of 15 mg/ml seems to be necessary in order to provide good operating conditions (Liu SS, personal communication). For some procedures, a dose of 40 mg may be adequate,[19] but in most cases a dose of 50–70 mg would be more reliable. In our institution, we use 20 mg/ml hyperbaric solution. This will still cause some TNS cases but no cases of PNTD have been reported so far.

Mepivacaine, procaine, chloroprocaine, prilocaine
These drugs are not very well studied and documented for spinal anaesthesia, but as the incidence of TNS is lower than with lidocaine and the duration of action comparable, they are interesting alternatives. Due to limited use for spinal anaesthesia, it is hard to say whether these drugs are less associated with PNTD than lidocaine. Whereas procaine is too short lasting and chloroprocaine causes a high incidence of backache, prilocaine

seems promising, with reliable anaesthesia lasting 20–40% longer than lido-caine in similar doses and a lower rate of TNS.

Bupivacaine
In small doses,[17] eventually combined with spinal adjuvants,[18] bupivacaine may have a short clinical duration of action, comparable to lidocaine. However, there are data which indicate that the paralysing effects of bupiva-caine on the detrusor muscles are still prolonged, increasing the risk of unwarranted catheterisation compared with lidocaine.[20]

Pethidine (meperidine)
Pethidine has been suggested as an interesting alternative to the pure local anaesthetics. It acts both as a local anaesthetic and as an opioid, thus using a multimodal principle which may lower the dose and reduce the incidence of side effects.[21] A dose of 40–50 mg may give efficient anaesthesia for surgery of 1–2 hours duration with extended postoperative pain relief for 15 hours afterwards.[22] However, as with all spinal opioids, the side effects may be nausea, pruritus, urinary retention, and respiratory depression.

Adjuvants
A variety of adjuvants have been used with spinal anaesthesia, including opioids, α_2 agonists and, more experimentally, neostigmine. The role of neostigmine is still questioned. While providing reliable adjuvant analgesia, it is also a potent emetic agent if the dose is too high or the cephalad spread too extensive.[23] Epinephrine may intensify and prolong the duration of spinal local anaesthetics, but it has been shown that the ability to void and discharge may be delayed more than the prolongation of anaesthesia.[24] Opioids, however, are valuable adjuvants in order to decrease the dose of local anaesthetic drug without prolonging recovery.[25] However, it is important to limit the dose in order to avoid respiratory depression; 10–25 µg of fentanyl may seem appropriate.[25] However, a more than 50% rate of pruritus may still be encountered.[25]

Another approach to minimise the spinal anaesthetic dose is to have an epidural catheter in place for top-ups in those cases where a minimum dose turns out to be insufficient. Urmey and colleagues report the successful use of lidocaine 40 mg to produce spinal anaesthesia lasting for 1–1.5 hours, combined with an epidural catheter and top-ups when needed.[19]

Practical spinal technique

Lidocaine is still the drug of choice when a short-acting spinal anaesthetic is needed. In a 2% solution and doses in the 40–70 mg range, no permanent nerve tissue damage has been reported. However, prilocaine should be tested more extensively in order to elucidate its role as a less TNS-provoking alternative to lidocaine. In very short cases or where rapid postoperative mobilisation is essential, the lidocaine dose (and thus the duration of anaesthesia) may be kept at a minimum with an adjuvant of 10 μg of fentanyl, intravenous or inhalational adjuvants or an epidural catheter as a rescue. Whereas TNS is a benign and self-limiting condition, it may have an unacceptably high incidence after lidocaine for procedures in the lithotomy position or after knee arthroscopy. In these cases a low dose of bupivacaine (e.g. 5–10 mg) may be an alternative, possibly with fentanyl added, although a risk of delayed discharge due to late voiding may be a problem.

A practical technique is summarised in Box 5.2. My choice is to have the patient sitting on the operating table with their head flexed. I use a 27 G

Box 5.2 Summary of spinal anaesthesia (see text for full details)

Suitable procedures:	Perineal and lower body procedures
Landmarks:	L2–3 or L3–4 interspace in midline; 27 G Whitacre needle
Endpoint:	Flow back of cerebrospinal fluid
Local anaesthetic:	3–3.5 ml 2% lidocaine in 7.5% glucose
	(3 ml 0.25% bupivacaine in 4% glucose ± fentanyl, 10 μg)
Onset:	2–3 min (≈ 10 min with bupivacaine)
Duration:	1–3 h
Comments:	Preload with 250–500 ml saline
	Keep patient sitting up for 2 min for perineal procedures

Whittacre needle with introducer in the L2–3 or L3–4 interspace in the midline. After spinal backflow, I inject 60–70 mg of lidocaine 20 mg/ml in 7.5% glucose (hyperbaric), withdraw the needle and lay the patient supine. In the case of a perineal operation, I will let the patient sit for 2 minutes before positioning him or her on the table.

Brachial plexus anaesthesia[26]

Whereas the supraclavicular approach is discouraged in ambulatory practice due to the danger of pneumothorax, the axillary approach may be recommended for all procedures in the elbow, lower arm, hand or fingers. With a proper technique, a tourniquet on the upper arm will also be well accepted. The drawback with axillary block, as with all methods of brachial plexus block, is the risk of failure which, even in experienced hands, has a 5–10% incidence. Furthermore, the dose required is on the limit of toxic potential and the risk of inadvertent IV injection or rapid vascular absorption is higher than with most other regional techniques. In order to minimise these problems, a dedicated regimen should be used for axillary plexus block. Due to a high background failure rate, many alternative regimens exist.

Practical brachial plexus technique

This technique is summarised in Box 5.3 and the anatomy is illustrated in

Box 5.3 Summary of axillary brachial plexus block. (see text for full details)

Suitable procedures:	Upper limb operations from elbow down
Landmarks:	Palpation of artery high in axilla; 23 G sharp needle
Endpoint:	Paraesthesia (or response at ≤0.5 mA) prior to arterial puncture
	Puncture artery then advance needle until no blood aspirated
Local anaesthetic:	Mix 20 ml 2% lidocaine with 12.5 µg/ml epinephrine, 20 ml 1% lidocaine plain (or 20 ml each of 1% and 2% both with 5 µg/ml epinephrine) and 10 ml saline
	If paraesthesia elicited, inject 25 ml and remainder beyond artery; if artery punctured first, inject all 50 ml beyond artery
Onset:	15–30 min
Duration:	2–4 h (8–10 h if 1% lidocaine replaced with 0.5% bupivacaine)
Comments:	Apply distal compression for 2 min with arm adducted

Figure 5.1. I use 50 ml of lidocaine at a concentration of 12 mg/ml, containing 4–6 µg/ml epinephrine. This can be achieved by mixing suitable commercial preparations, depending upon what is locally available. One option is 20 ml of lidocaine 20 mg/ml with epinephrine 12.5 µg/ml, 20 ml of 10 mg/ml lidocaine plain and 10 ml saline. Alternatively, 20 ml of lidocaine 20 mg/ml and 20 ml of lidocaine 10 mg/ml, each with epinephrine 5 µg/ml, plus 10 ml saline is also suitable. For an adult, all 50 ml will be injected as high in the axilla as possible, with a distal compression for two minutes afterwards with the arm adducted. A high volume is important in order to increase the success rate and, together with a proximal injection, minimises any discomfort from a tourniquet. I use a 23 G sharp needle, with a short extension line to the syringe (Fig. 5.2), aiming for the axillary artery with the needle. If I hit the artery, I will penetrate to the posterior side (i.e. no more fresh red aspirate) and deposit 50 ml of the local anaesthetic solution slowly, with frequent attempts at aspiration in order to avoid intraarterial injection. If paraesthesia is elicited before entering the artery, I

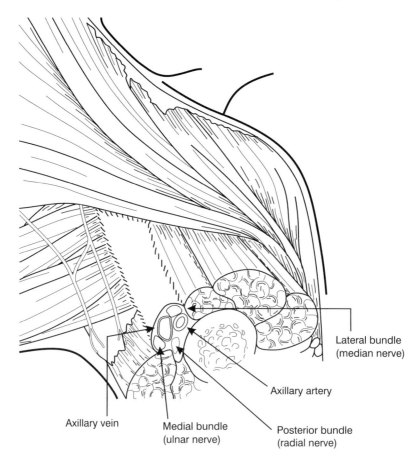

Figure 5.1 The anatomy of the brachial plexus in the axilla. The left side is illustrated.

withdraw the needle 1 mm and then inject 25 ml of the solution while asking the patient if there is any radiating pain which, if present, calls for a further withdrawal of the needle. The residual 25 ml I try to put transarterially (see above). If it is not important to fully block the radial nerve, I first try to hit (i.e. elicit paraesthesia in) the nerve bundle medial to the artery for an ulnar nerve block and the bundle lateral to the artery for a median nerve block.

For the trainee, a nerve stimulator will be helpful, using the same landmarks as above, using 3 mA at the start, reduced to 1 mA when a nerve response is present and then not injecting until a response is still present at 0.5 mA or lower. The nerve stimulator technique is less traumatic and slightly less painful for the patient, but is more expensive and takes more time. It may still end in failure, because the response may be elicited through the connective tissue sheet surrounding the nerve bundle. Thus, the injection may be on the outside of this sheet with insufficient effect, in spite of a good nerve stimulator response.

Whereas a lidocaine block in the axilla will provide surgical anaesthesia within 15–30 minutes which lasts for 2–4 hours, an alternative is to mix 20 ml of bupivacaine 5 mg/ml instead of the lidocaine 10 mg/ml in the recipe above. The onset of anaesthesia will be about the same, but the duration of the block may be 8–10 hours. This may be appropriate if significant postoperative pain is expected, but the patient should be instructed to use a sling and to be careful with their paralysed arm after discharge.

Interscalene block[26]

This block is appropriate for shoulder surgery, arthroscopy, and upper arm surgery. The lower arm and hand are often not adequately anaesthetised, especially the area supplied by the ulnar nerve. It is important to realise that this block almost invariably results in diaphragmatic hemiparesis and should be used with caution in patients with pulmonary disease who are dependent upon optimal diaphragmatic function. Bilateral block should not be attempted. Some patients may also have a Horner's syndrome with this

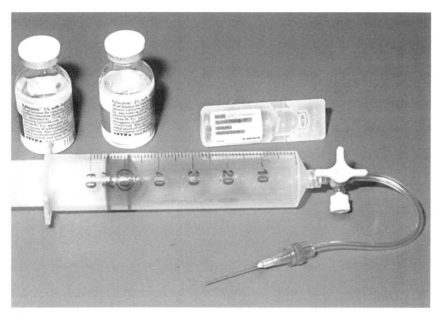

Figure 5.2 Equipment for performing brachial plexus block. Twenty ml of each local anaesthetic solution is mixed with 10 ml saline to give a total volume of 50 ml. This is injected using a 23 G sharp needle attached to a short extension (the three-way tap is unnecessary but comes as an integral part of the extension used here).

block.

The drug mixture and equipment will be identical to that used during axillary block (see above, Figure 5.2). The patient should lie with a towel under the shoulder, in order to stretch the neck and slightly rotate the head against the healthy upper extremity. A short cough or head lift may help to visualise the interscalene groove, just lateral to the middle of the sternocleidomastoid muscle (Figure 5.3). From a position behind the patient's head, a 23 G needle (attached to a nerve stimulator) should be advanced downward and backward into the scalene groove until paraesthesia or jerks in the shoulder muscles are elicited. A slow injection of 30–35 ml of anaesthetic solution (see above), with frequent aspiration and no radiating pain, will be sufficient for a reliable block.

Intravenous regional anaesthesia

This technique is easy to learn and use and administration is rapid. A double tourniquet is applied to the upper arm. Even with the use of this double tourniquet, there will be some discomfort from the tourniquet,

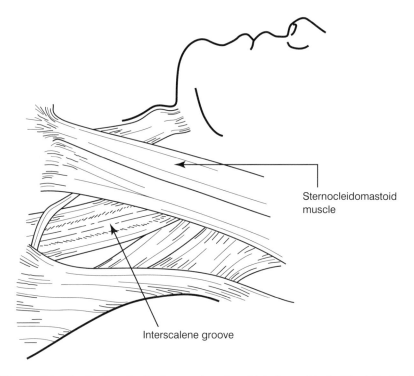

Sternocleidomastoid muscle

Interscalene groove

Figure 5.3 The landmarks for interscalene brachial plexus block. The left side is drawn.

which limits the recommended duration of the surgical procedure to a maximum of 45–60 minutes. The block is most successful with superficial procedures or operations involving soft tissues, whereas bones or joints may not be adequately anaesthetised. Inadequate block may be obtained in obese individuals and, of course, if for some reason the cuff is leaking.

The technique is to insert a thin (0.8 or 1.0 mm) IV cannula into a vein on the hand, to squeeze the blood out of the arm with an elastic, rubber bandage and to inflate the proximal cuff with a pressure of 100–150 mmHg above the systolic pressure. Then the rubber band is released and 40 ml of lidocaine 5 mg/ml without epinephrine is injected through the IV line. After the lidocaine is distributed (3–5 minutes) the distal cuff is inflated and the proximal is released. This cuff should never be released until at least 15–20 minutes has passed, because of the danger of toxic symptoms from rapid access of high-dose local anaesthetics into the circulation. For the same reason, bupivacaine is not recommended for this block at all and in the UK, prilocaine is the preferred choice. After 20 minutes, much of the lidocaine will be bound to tissue and at cuff deflation the release of drug into circulation will be somewhat slowed, usually not causing any generalised symptoms. For safety, an IV cannula should always be placed in the contralateral arm prior to block placement.

Epidural anaesthesia

Whereas spinal anaesthesia is frequently used for day case anaesthesia,[8] epidural anaesthesia has some drawbacks. In particular, it is more time consuming to administer and there is a delay in onset of the block.

However, there are situations where an epidural block may be appropriate. Some patients may have had a bad previous experience with spinal headache or fear this complication. Some female patients may have had good experiences with epidural anaesthesia during childbirth and may request the same method again. Some surgical procedures may have an unpredictable or long duration, so the flexibility of extra dosing through an epidural catheter may be important. Examples are knee arthroscopy, which sometimes may turn in to extensive cruciate ligament repair, or prolonged procedures for varicose veins or plastic surgery in the lower half of the body.[27]

Minimising the drawbacks of epidural anaesthesia

The main focus in this respect is to limit the time taken by epidural anaesthesia, both for the anaesthetist and especially to avoid delays for the rest of the perioperative team. Some practical aspects must be addressed, in particular the choice of local anaesthetic drug.

Drugs of long duration are not appropriate because most ambulatory surgical procedures take less than 1–2 hours and, if they last longer, top-up doses of a short-acting agent through the epidural catheter work well. Prolonged epidural anaesthesia may result in extended postoperative bed occupancy, delayed discharge, and increased risk of urinary retention.[8] Thus ropivacaine or bupivacaine are usually not recommended, except in children.[28]

In adults, lidocaine seems to be the drug of choice for epidural anaesthesia in day cases.[29] It has a fairly fast onset and intermediate duration, a low cardiotoxicity and is extensively documented. In order to speed up the onset, lower the systemic absorption and increase the anaesthetic potency of lidocaine, the addition of a small amount of epinephrine (5–10 μg/ml) is recommended.[8] Other measures to speed up the onset of block with lidocaine are to add 0.5 mmol of bicarbonate per 10 ml injected or to use lidocaine warmed to body temperature instead of using the drug directly from the refrigerator.[8]

Due to the need for prolonged postoperative surveillance, the use of morphine in the epidural mixture is usually not recommended in day surgery. Some authors have recently advocated the use of short-acting opioids (e.g. alfentanil, fentanyl, sufentanil) in order to speed up the onset, improve the quality of the block and improve postoperative analgesia. In a study by Kwa and co-workers, the addition of sufentanil 0.5 μg/ml to a 5 mg/ml solution of lidocaine with epinephrine had an onset of six minutes and was fully adequate for surgery.[30]

Practical epidural administration

Some preloading (i.e. 250–500 ml) with an IV electrolyte or colloid infusion is beneficial and should preferably be done in the preoperative holding area in order not to occupy the operating theatre for longer than necessary. For the same reason, it may be very useful to perform the epidural block in the holding area or in an induction room if that is practical and compatible with general guidelines for the safety of epidural anaesthesia. For the purpose of preventing hypotension and associated nausea, the early use of ephedrine is probably more efficient than wasting time on extensive preloading.

A small amount of local anaesthetic should be used with a thin needle to anaesthetise the skin in the appropriate level before an 18 G or thinner epidural needle is introduced. My favourite is to use the loss of resistance technique with saline and the lateral decubitus patient position, but with obese patients a sitting position is often easier to succeed with.

Some controversial issues are the use of a catheter, the use of a test dose and whether we insert the catheter before or after injecting the full dose. The first issue is least controversial; the versatility of epidural anaesthesia is lost without the catheter, and apart from occasional tearing of blood vessels and mild paraesthesias, there are few drawbacks to inserting a catheter.

The other issues are more controversial and are interlinked. What we do not want is an occasional very high dose delivered spinally through an epidural tear or an inadvertent intravenous injection of a large dose of local anaesthetic drug, resulting in a possible cerebral or cardiovascular toxic reaction. The problem with the test dose is that, even with a fairly high specificity and sensitivity in order to detect a subarachnoid injection, this situation is so rare in experienced hands that the chance of false-positive or negative test dose results may be 5–10 times higher than a true-positive result. This has led many authorities to conclude that in experienced hands, a test dose is not recommended (Scott B and Mulroy M, personal communication). If the test dose is given through the needle, there is the risk that the patient may move with the needle in situ while waiting to observe the effects of the test dose. Therefore, a test dose should still be used after the catheter is placed, since the catheter itself may tear a vein or the dura during insertion. Thus, most of those advocating a test dose conclude that it is most appropriately used after the catheter has been introduced.

If the full dose is injected slowly, before introducing the epidural catheter, it will open up the epidural space in a dissecting way, which will probably reduce the chance of tearing a vessel when introducing the catheter. The vessel may more easily slip away from the catheter tip when floating free in a widened epidural space, compared with the firm attachment to neighbouring structures if only a small injection into the epidural space has taken place. However, while the test dose may be unreliable, that does not mean that it is safe to inject a full dose of epidural anaesthetic directly. Some issues are still important. Inject slowly, over at least two minutes; use 14–16 ml lidocaine at 15 mg/ml with 5–10 μg/ml of epinephrine and inject through the needle. In the event of an accidental spinal tap, the warm flow of fluid out of the needle is readily felt before the syringe is attached. Furthermore, symptoms of a spinal anaesthetic generally appear within 30 seconds, therefore stopping injecting at this point will probably produce no more than a slightly overdosed spinal anaesthetic, at worst. A spinal overdose is also treatable without sequelae, should it occur. In a worst-case scenario, where the full dose has been intravenously administered over two minutes, there should still be no permanent harm, even if convulsions occur. Such a dose of 4 mg/kg may result in a serum concentration in the lower range for cerebral convulsions (8–12 mg/l), but with lidocaine this is well below cardiac toxicity levels.[31] The α half-life of lidocaine is 2–4 minutes, thus with a slow injection much of the drug is cleared from serum during administration, further reducing the risk of convulsions.

Perioperative aspects

As previously mentioned, placing the epidural before entering the operating theatre if possible is beneficial. Otherwise, in experienced hands there should be no need to wait for the full effect of the block before allowing the scrub nurse to begin preparation of the patient. Thus, if the block has to be placed in the operating theatre, the nurses should go ahead shortly after the epidural catheter is in place. In some countries, these nursing preparations may take 15–20 minutes or more, in which case the use of an appropriate epidural technique may not delay the start of the operation significantly. The only reason to wait for the effect of the block before washing and draping is in the case of block failure. In experienced hands, epidural block failure rates should be less than a few percent and in those rare cases, a rescue general anaesthetic should be introduced after the draping of the patient, when the block failure is confirmed.

An alternative in order to avoid preoperative delay is to use the combination of spinal and epidural anaesthesia (CSE). Special needle kits are available for this combination through a single skin insertion (e.g. spinal through epidural needle), but the method may also be practised with an ordinary spinal injection followed with a separate epidural catheter insertion.

Hypotension should be prevented by some volume preloading, but care should be taken not to give more than 1–1.5 litres of saline solutions, unless the patient has a significant blood loss. Extensive fluid loading may result in increased need for urinary catheterisation, due to either bladder filling or urinary retention.[8] Transient head-down position and liberal use of ephedrine are appropriate measures if hypotension does occur.

Box 5.4 Summary of epidural anaesthesia (see text for full details)

Suitable procedures:	Lower body operations of variable (possibly long) duration
Landmarks:	L2–3 or L3–4 interspace in midline; 18 G Tuhoy needle
Endpoint:	Loss of resistance to air or saline
Local anaesthetic:	Mix 10 ml 2% lidocaine with 12.5 µg/ml epinephrine and 10 ml 1% plain lidocaine (or 10 ml each of 1% and 2% both with 5 µg/ml epinephrine). Inject 1–2 ml into skin and 14–16 ml through *needle* over 2–3 min
Onset:	15–30 min. Inject further 5–10 ml if poor block after 5–10 min
Duration:	1–2 h, but can top up with 6–8 ml/h
Comments:	Preload with 250–500 ml saline

Practical epidural technique

I consider the use of epidural anaesthesia for day case surgery on the lower half of the body if the operation is expected to be prolonged for more than two hours, if the extension of surgery is very unpredictable or if there is a special request from the patient. The technique is summarised in Box 5.4. I mix 50:50 the two commercial solutions of lidocaine, 20 mg/ml with epinephrine 12.5 µg/ml and 10 mg/ml plain (or 10 ml each of 1% and 2% both with 5 µg/ml epinephrine), use 1–2 ml for skin anaesthesia and 14–16 ml for injection over 2–3 minutes through the epidural needle. I check for a dural tap before the start of injection, carefully aspirate and look for blood during the injection and continuously talk to the patient during the injection and ask them to report any numbness in the buttocks or lower limbs or any sensation of changes in taste, vision or other cranial nerve symptoms. After injection, I slowly advance the catheter 2 cm into the epidural space, secure it and place the patient on the table ready for washing and draping. After 8–10 minutes I inject a further 5–10 ml through the catheter if there are signs of too slow development of the block or if the level of anaesthesia needs to be above the T10–12 level.

Just before the start of surgery, I ask the patient to describe the sensation in their legs and ask the assistant nurse or the surgeon to carefully test for pain at the operation site. If the procedure takes more than two hours, I will top up the epidural with 6–8 ml/h of the initial lidocaine mixture after one hour and then hourly.

Caudal epidural block in children

Although children mostly do not want to have regional blocks or be awake during surgery and most blocks are not recommended under deep general anaesthesia (see above), the caudal epidural technique is very useful to reduce anaesthetic requirements and to provide superior postoperative pain relief. In contrast to adults, children may be discharged with caudal epidural block still working, because they do not have any risk of haemodynamic instability during offset of the block and they do not get urinary retention.[8]

Children may therefore benefit from the choice of a long-acting epidural block in day case surgery, due to effective postoperative pain relief with a very low incidence of nausea. Due to less cardiotoxicity and slightly less motor block, ropivacaine would seem preferable to bupivacaine for caudal blocks in children. With a 2 mg/ml solution without epinephrine, 0.75 ml/kg may be used for perineal surgery, whereas 1–1.5 ml/kg is appropriate for hernia repair and surgery in the external genital area. A maximum dose of 20 ml is to be observed.

My technique is to have the anaesthetised child on their side with knees, hips, and head flexed. With a 23 G needle, an extension line and a 10 ml syringe, I go into the sacral hiatus, feel the click on entering the dura, stop without advancing further, aspirate and then slowly inject ropivacaine while aspirating regularly.

Box 5.5 Summary of caudal epidural anaesthesia in children (see text for full details)

Suitable procedures:	Perineal, genital or inguinal surgery in children
Landmarks:	Sacral hiatus in anaesthetised child; 23 G needle and extension
Endpoint:	Click upon dural puncture; free aspiration of air
Local anaesthetic:	Plain ropivacaine 2 mg/ml. 0.75 ml/kg for perineal surgery, 1–1.5 ml/kg for inguinal/genital surgery
Onset:	10–15 min
Duration:	3–6 h (individual and dose dependent)
Comments:	Maximum volume 20 ml

Paracervical block

This is an easy block to perform with a rapid onset (within 3–5 minutes) and gives good anaesthesia for uterine dilatation and curettage and for hysteroscopy. It is an excellent alternative to general anaesthesia in obese patients and patients with a minor upper airway infection. It is usually most practical for the gynaecologist to administer the block; 10 ml of lidocaine 10 mg/ml with epinephrine on each side. There is a risk of intravenous injection in the highly vascularised uterine tissue and some patient discomfort may be present if the uterus is vigorously manipulated.

Inguinal hernia block

With an appropriate technique (Box 5.6), this block provides excellent surgical and postoperative analgesia for hernia repair, simplifying the anaesthetic management and postoperative care compared to either general or spinal anaesthesia. A blunt needle should be inserted 2 cm medial to the anterior superior tubercle of the iliac crest (Figure 5.4). The needle is advanced slowly and a 7 ml dose of lidocaine 10 mg/ml is administered after achieving a loss of resistance. The needle is then advanced 0.5–1 cm and a further 7 ml given after detecting a second loss of resistance. A spinal needle should then be used to infiltrate the skin area for the wound with another 10–15 ml. Finally, a blunt needle should be used 1 cm cephalad to the midpoint of the inguinal ligament, going deep subfascially and injecting a further 20–25 ml. The subfascial position is confirmed when a second click is felt as the blunt needle is advanced slowly into the layers, starting from the skin.

Box 5.6 Summary of inguinal hernia block (see text for full details)

Suitable procedures:	Inguinal hernia repair
Landmarks:	1) 2 cm medial to anterior superior tubercle of iliac crest
	2) 1 cm cephalad to midpoint of inguinal ligament
Endpoint:	1) Click after penetrating oblique muscles
	2) Second click deep to fascia
Local anaesthetic:	1% plain lidocaine. 7 ml at point (1); 20–25 ml deep at point (2); 10–15 ml *via* spinal needle along line of incision
Onset:	5–10 min
Duration	2–3 h

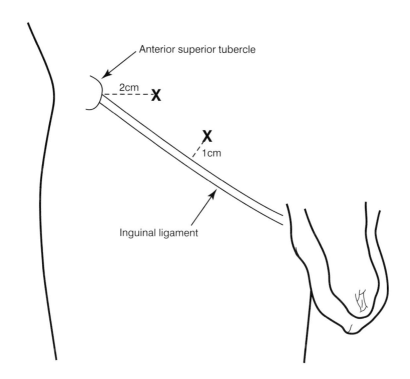

Figure 5.4 The landmarks for performing a regional block for right inguinal hernia repair. Injections are made 2 cm medial to the anterior superior tubercle of the iliac crest and 1 cm cephalad to the midpoint of the inguinal ligament.

Femoral block[32]

This is a simple block which may be useful for knee surgery, either as an adjunct to local anaesthesia in the knee joint, to general anaesthesia or together with the sciatic nerve block for a fully anaesthetised lower limb. Twenty ml of lidocaine 10 mg/ml with epinephrine may be injected in a fan-like fashion 0.5–3 cm lateral to the femoral artery. A more extended block which also includes the obturator and lateral cutaneous femoral nerve may be accomplished with the three-in-one technique. For this block, the needle should be advanced somewhat deeper and proximal under the inguinal ligament and, after eliciting paraesthesia (or muscle jerks with a nerve stimulator), a dose of 40 ml should be injected slowly.

Sciatic nerve block[32]

This block is a useful alternative, together with a femoral block, if only one leg needs to be anaesthetised. The patient should lie on their side with the hips flexed 45°. A line between the femoral trochanter and the superior posterior iliac spine should be drawn (Fig. 5.5) and 4–5 cm distal to the middle of this line paraesthesia should be sought, using a spinal needle. Twenty ml of lidocaine 10 mg/ml with epinephrine should be administered.

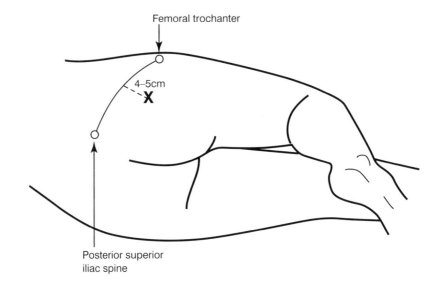

Figure 5.5 The landmarks for sciatic nerve block on the right-hand side. The line joins the femoral trochanter and the superior posterior iliac spine and an injection is made 4–5 cm distal to the middle of this line, after eliciting paraesthesia.

Ankle Block

This is a very useful block for all kind of procedures in the foot. As the block is somewhat painful, it may be advisable to give the patient a small dose of an opioid (e.g. alfentanil 0.5 mg IV) before starting. The anatomy is illustrated in Figure 5.6. My choice is to use a 23 G needle, first going behind the medial malleolus, behind the artery, searching for paraesthesia down in the foot. Once paraesthesia is found, withdraw for 1 mm, aspirate and inject 5–7 ml of lidocaine 20 mg/ml with epinephrine. Then, I change to a 10 ml

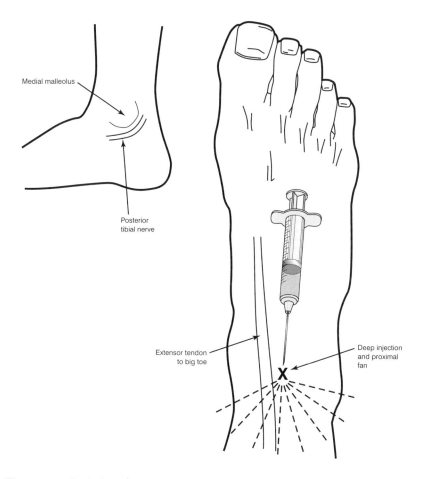

Figure 5.6 Technique for ankle block in the right foot. The first injection is made when paraesthesia is elicited at a point behind the medial malleolus and posterior tibial artery. The second injection is made deep, lateral to the extensor muscle of the big toe, from where a medial and lateral semicircular subcutaneous cuff is fanned out in front of the distal leg.

syringe with lidocaine 10 mg/ml without epinephrine and inject 2 ml deep, lateral to the extensor tendon of the big toe. Then I use the needle from the same injection in a fan, both medially and laterally, making a semicircular subcutaneous cuff in front of the distal leg, proximal to the malleoli, injecting 8–12 ml of local anaesthetic. The benefit of this technique is that the fan both relieves the pain of a distal tourniquet and provides analgesia in the dorsum of the foot. If prolonged postoperative analgesia is required for 10–12 hours, the lidocaine may be replaced with bupivacaine 2.5 or 5.0 mg/ml respectively. This technique is summarised in Box 5.7.

Box 5.7 Summary of ankle block (see text for full details)

Suitable procedures:	All foot operations
Landmarks:	1) Behind artery behind medial malleolus
	2) Lateral to the extensor tendon of the big toe
Endpoint:	1) Paraesthesia going down foot
Local anaesthetic:	1) 5–7 ml 2% lidocaine with epinephrine
	2) 2 ml 1% plain lidocaine, deep. Continue to fan out medially and laterally, inject a subcutaneous cuff in front of leg; 8–12 ml
Onset:	5–10 min
Duration:	4–6 h (10–12 h using 0.25% or 0.5% bupivacaine)
Comments:	Painful block, may require IV opioid analgesia

Summary

A considerable proportion of all day case surgical procedures may be performed under regional anaesthesia. Most of the techniques are relatively simple to learn and perform, are effective in most patients and do not introduce significant delays once the anaesthetist has become reasonably experienced. Patients and surgeons may initially be reluctant to embrace regional anaesthesia, but once this practice is adopted, it is generally well received. For the patient, regional anaesthesia offers good perioperative analgesia, rapid and clear-headed recovery without the nausea and somnolence associated with general anaesthesia and the opportunity to see the intraoperative findings for themselves. For the surgeon and anaesthetist, there is the benefit of a cooperative and responsive patient and, for the day surgery unit, the opportunity to reduce direct drug costs and minimise the use of the phase I recovery unit.

A great number of regional anaesthetic blocks have been described and variations of technique exist for many of these. Nevertheless, just a small selection of blocks will be sufficient for the majority of procedures routinely encountered. Regional anaesthesia is not without its problems and serious complications sometimes occur. For some procedures, residual sympathetic and motor block may delay discharge in comparison to general anaesthesia. Many regional anaesthetic procedures are initially painful and there is an ever-present failure rate. No technique is perfect, however, and with careful attention to detail, appropriate choice of local anaesthetic agent and dose and the use of adjuvant analgesia and sedation where necessary, most of these problems can be minimised. Regional anaesthesia is not suitable for all patients and procedures but its use should probably be more widespread than it currently is in many day surgery units.

1   Dahl JB, Kehlet H. The value of pre-emptive analgesia in the treatment of postoperative pain (Review). *Br J Anaesth* 1993;**70**:434–9.
2   Warner MA, Shields SE, Chute CG. Major morbidity and mortality within 1 month of ambulatory surgery and anesthesia. *JAMA* 1993;**270**:1437–41.
3   Kroll DA, Caplan RA, Posner K, Ward RJ, Cheney FW. Nerve injury associated with anesthesia. *Anesthesiology* 1990;**73**:202–7.
4   Cheney FW. The American Society of Anesthesiologists closed claims project. *Anesthesiology* 1999;**91**:552–6.
5   Scug S. The CORTRA study. A collaborative overview of randomized trials of regional anaesthesia. In: Winnie AP, ed. *Highlights in regional anaesthesia and pain therapy*. Cyprus: ESRA, 1999:177–9.
6   Moller JT, Cluitmans P, Rasmussen LS *et al.* Long-term postoperative cognitive dysfunction in the elderly: ISPOCD1 study. International Study of Post-Operative Cognitive Dysfunction. *Lancet* 1998;**351**:857–61.
7   Dahl V, Gierloff C, Omland E, Ræder JC. Spinal, epidural or propofol anaesthesia for out-patient knee arthroscopy? *Acta Anaesthesiol Scand* 1997;**41**:1341–5.
8   Ræder JC, Korttila K. Regional anaesthesia for day surgery. In: Prys-Roberts C, Brown BRJ, eds. *International practice of anaesthesia*. Oxford: Butterworth-Heinemann, 1996:1–8.
9   Bordahl PE, Ræder JC, Nordentoft J, Kirste U, Refsdal A. Laparoscopic sterilization under local or general anesthesia? A randomized study. *Obs Gynecol* 1993;**81**:137–41.
10 Wulf H. Epidural anaesthesia and spinal haematoma. *Can J Anaesth* 1996;**43**:1260–71.
11 Drolet P, Veillette Y. Back pain following epidural anesthesia with 2-chloroprocaine (EDTA-free) or lidocaine. *Reg Anesth* 1997;**22**:303–7.
12 Hiller A, Rosenberg PH. Transient neurological symptoms after spinal anaesthesia with 4% mepivacaine and 0.5% bupivacaine. *Br J Anaesth* 1997;**79**:301–5.
13 Kubina P, Gupta A, Oscarsson A, Axelsson K, Bengtsson M. Two cases of cauda equina syndrome following spinal-epidural anesthesia. *Reg Anesth* 1997;**22**:447–50.
14 Pollock JE, Neal JM, Stephenson CA, Wiley CE. Prospective study of the incidence of transient radicular irritation in patients undergoing spinal anesthesia. *Anesthesiology* 1996;**84**:1361–7.
15 Loo CC, Irrestedt L. Cauda equina syndrome after spinal anaesthesia with hyperbaric 5% lignocaine: a review of six cases of cauda equina syndrome reported to the Swedish Pharmaceutical Insurance 1993–1997. *Acta Anaesthesiol Scand* 1999;**43**:371–9.
16 Liu SS. Drugs for spinal anesthesia: Past, present, and future (review). *Reg Anesth Pain Med* 1998;**23**:344–6.
17 Ben-David B, Levin H, Solomon E, Admoni H, Vaida S. Spinal bupivacaine in ambulatory surgery: the effect of saline dilution. *Anesth Analg* 1996;**83**:716–20.
18 Ben-David B, Solomon E, Levin H, Admoni H, Goldik Z. Intrathecal fentanyl with small-dose dilute bupivacaine: better anesthesia without prolonging recovery. *Anesth Analg* 1997;**85**:560–5.

19   Urmey WF, Stanton J, Peterson M, Sharrock NE. Combined spinal-epidural anesthesia for outpatient surgery. Dose-response characteristics of intrathecal isobaric lidocaine using a 27-gauge Whitacre spinal needle. *Anesthesiology* 1995;**83**:528–34.

20   Kamphuis ET, Ionescu TI, Kuipers PWG, de Gier J, van Venrooij GEPM, Boon TA. Recovery of storage and emptying functions of the urinary bladder after spinal anesthesia with lidocaine and with bupivacaine in men. *Anesthesiology* 1998;**88**:310–16.

21   Ngan Kee WD. Intrathecal pethidine: pharmacology and clinical applications (review). *Anaesth Intens Care* 1998;**26**:137–46.

22   Chaudhari LS, Kane DG, Shivkumar B, Kamath SK. Comparative study of intrathecal pethidine versus lignocaine as an anaesthetic and a postoperative analgesic for perianal surgery. *J Postgrad Med* 1996;**42**:43–5.

23   Pan PM, Huang CT, Wei TT, Mok MS. Enhancement of analgesic effect of intrathecal neostigmine and clonidine on bupivacaine spinal anesthesia. *Reg Anesth Pain Med* 1998;**23**:49–56.

24   Moore JM, Liu SS, Pollock JE, Neal JM, Knab JH. The effect of epinephrine on small-dose hyperbaric bupivacaine spinal anesthesia: clinical implications for ambulatory surgery. *Anesth Analg* 1998;**86**:973–7.

25   Chilvers CR, Vaghadia H, Mitchell GWE, Merrick PM. Small-dose hypobaric lidocaine-fentanyl spinal anesthesia for short duration outpatient laparoscopy. II. Optimal fentanyl dose. *Anesth Analg* 1997;**84**:65–70.

26   Winnie P. *Plexus anesthesia*. Fribourg: Mediglobe SA, 1993.

27   Knize DM, Fishell R. Use of preoperative subcutaneous "wetting solution" and epidural block anesthesia for liposuction in the office-based surgical suite. *Plast Reconstr Surg* 1997;**100**:1867–74.

28   Lawhorn CD, Stoner JM, Schmitz ML *et al.* Caudal epidural butorphanol plus bupivacaine versus bupivacaine in pediatric outpatient genitourinary procedures. *J Clin Anesth* 1997;**9**:103–8.

29   Kopacz DJ, Mulroy MF. Chloroprocaine and lidocaine decrease hospital stay and admission rate after outpatient epidural anesthesia. *Reg Anesth* 1990;**15**:19–25.

30   Kwa AM, Murray WB, Foster PA. Low dose epidural lidocaine/sufentanil is effective for outpatient lithotripsy. *Mid East J Anesthesiol* 1995;**13**:71–8.

31   Burrows FA, Lerman J, LeDez KM, Strong HA. Pharmacokinetics of lidocaine in children with congenital heart disease. *Can J Anaesth* 1991;**38**:196–200.

32   Scott DB. *Techniques of regional anaesthesia*. Fribourg: Mediglobe SA, 1989.

6: Sedation

GLENDA RUDKIN

Overview

Sedation anaesthesia is becoming more widely practised in day surgery. This is primarily due to the availability of new, short-acting drugs and improved delivery systems, increased patient acceptance and to a "new breed" of surgeons comfortable with performing surgery under local anaesthesia with sedation.

The term "sedation" encompasses the administration of a drug or drugs to provide amnesia, anxiolysis, analgesia, and hypnosis. Such medications may be used alone, to facilitate endoscopy and other uncomfortable procedures, or to supplement local infiltration or regional anaesthesia (see Chapter 5). As an adjuvant to local anaesthetic drugs, sedation techniques may increase patient acceptability, facilitate longer procedures and extend the range of operations which can be performed without general anaesthesia.

The use of sedative techniques for day case surgery varies considerably from country to country. In the United States, such an approach is common whereas in the United Kingdom, general anaesthesia is often preferred. Nevertheless, sedative techniques are generally safer and permit more rapid recovery compared to general anaesthesia and so their use should be encouraged. This chapter reviews the various indications for sedation and describes the components which make up the sedation triad. This forms the basis for the rational choice of adjuvant drugs and the pharmacology of the more commonly used medications is discussed, with particular reference to sedative doses.

Although patient selection and recovery are more fully discussed elsewhere (Chapters 1 and 8), the key points relative to sedated patients are reviewed here. Finally this chapter will discuss some newer developments, some of which are still at the experimental stage, such as patient-controlled sedation, patient-maintained target-controlled sedation, and the use of anaesthetic depth monitors to guide sedation.

Definitions and terminology

Sedation for diagnostic and surgical procedures includes the administration, by any route or technique, of drugs which result in depression of the central nervous system. The objective is to produce a level of sedation where the patient is relaxed and has the ability to maintain an airway and respond appropriately to verbal communication.

Various terminologies have been used to describe sedation, such as conscious sedation, sedoanalgesia, monitored anaesthesia care (MAC) and neuroleptanalgesia. The practice of neuroleptanalgesia is now largely obsolete[1]. This term refers to the combination of a neuroleptic drug, such as haloperidol (butyrophenone) or droperidol, and an opioid, sometimes with the addition of nitrous oxide. The neurolept approach produces a state of indifference and immobilisation, being quite different to the minimally depressed state of consciousness which we will subsequently refer to as sedation. With the recent introduction of short-acting anxiolytics, hypnotics and analgesics, we are more able to provide a tailored sedative technique to suit fluctuating surgical demands and patient requirements.

The sedation triad

Why do we sedate patients? The objective is to produce a level of sedation where the patient is calm and relaxed but where rational verbal communication is continuously possible. There are three components to the sedation triad: anxiolysis, amnesia, and analgesia, which result in balanced sedation (Figure 6.1).

Depending upon the surgical procedure to be undertaken and the patient's request, different combinations and varying proportions of drugs are selected to meet the sedation triad requirements.[2] It may be that the patient wants to be drowsy but would like to recall events at surgery, in which case the potent amnesic drug, midazolam, would be avoided. Total analgesia may be achieved with local or regional anaesthesia techniques, so the addition of an opioid is unnecessary. However, during endoscopic

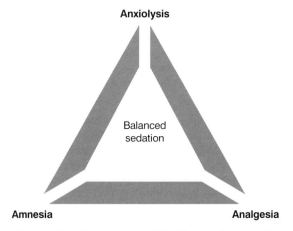

Figure 6.1 Components of the "triad of sedation"

procedures such as colonoscopy, the addition of an opioid will greatly enhance the quality of sedation, as pressure and traction are painful stimuli.

Pain, anxiety, and amnesia should be treated separately with the appropriate drug. The appropriate dose of all medications is titrated to the desired effect or, alternatively, patients may be allowed to titrate the drug themselves to their own needs, using the technique of patient-controlled sedation.

The necessity and extent of drug treatment can be minimised by thorough preoperative preparation and attention to the patient's specific needs. Patient comfort will also be assisted by supportive non-therapeutic measures (Box 6.1). Koch and colleagues have recently shown that intraoperative music has a calming effect in awake patients, potent enough to decrease their sedative and analgesic requirements.[3]

Box 6.1 Non-therapeutic measures to assist patient comfort and minimise drug requirements

- Warm operating atmosphere
- Warm infusion fluids
- Warm blankets
- Pillows and padding
- Soft mattress
- Posturing to suit patient needs
- Screening patient from surgery
- Music
    - Patient personal headphones
    - Patient choice
- Minimise operating theatre noise

There are significant advantages of sedation anaesthesia to the patient, the surgeon (or endoscopist) and to the day surgery facility (Box 6.2).

Box 6.2 Advantages to sedation anaesthesia

Patient advantages:	Reduced anxiety
	Tolerance to long procedures
	Avoidance of general anaesthesia risks
	Decreased postoperative pain
	Decreased postoperative nausea and vomiting
	Earlier ambulation and discharge
Surgeon advantages:	Optimal operating conditions
	Reduced operating times
	Reduced sympathetic response to surgery
	Discuss operative findings at surgery
Day surgery facility advantages	Costs reduced

Patient assessment

Comprehensive preoperative patient assessment is as important for patients undergoing sedation anaesthesia with regional or local anaesthesia as it is for those undergoing general anaesthesia. A practical streamlined system is outlined in Figure 6.2.

The assessment process can be streamlined by the use of a health questionnaire, which the preadmission registered nurse completes with the

---

Surgical consulation

- Encourages sedation anaesthesia for suitable procedure
- Patient given printed information regarding anaesthesia options

---

Assesment by preadmission registered nurse

- Identifies "at-risk" patient
- Refers "at-risk" patient to anaesthetist
- Reinforces verbal and written anaesthesia information
- Instructional sedation video shown
- Answers patient's questions and allays anxieties

Day of surgery assessment by anaesthetist

- Expectations and concerns discussed
- Choice of sedation *versus* general anaesthesia offered
- Informed consent

Figure 6.2 Flow chart for streamlined selection of patients who will undergo sedation anaesthesia.

patient. This will help identify "at-risk" patients preoperatively, generally ASA III or IV patients (Box 6.3). The anaesthetist should take additional care in monitoring "at-risk" patients, selecting and titrating appropriate drugs and thereby avoiding complications.

Box 6.3 Patient groups considered especially "at risk" for day case surgery

- Elderly
- Morbidly obese
- History of sleep apnoea
- Mentally and neurologically handicapped
- Chronic respiratory disease
- Aspiration risk
- Medically unstable

Published surveys demonstrate that sedation techniques are considered to be most advantageous in the elderly and critically ill patients who are at greater risk from general anaesthetic complications.[4] With appropriate monitoring and surveillance, elderly patients pose no additional risk in the day surgery setting when administered sedative agents.[5]

Patient preparation

A fully informed patient who has received a thorough preoperative explanation will have less preoperative anxiety on the day of surgery and better rapport with their surgeon and anaesthetist. This will also assist the informed consent process.

Patients who are scheduled for sedation anaesthesia should be fasted according to general anaesthetic guidelines (see Chapter 1). This is important from a safety aspect, in case protective airway reflexes are lost or if general anaesthesia has to be administered. In the day surgery setting, premedication to allay anxiety is often unnecessary. Patient anxiety can be minimised by:

- full explanation about surgery and sedation anaesthesia before admission
- minimising preoperative waiting time
- a relaxing atmosphere
- provision of music by personal headphones.

Patient choices and sedation endpoints

The anaesthetist must consider individual patients' needs[6] and choices[7] for sedation. Sedation issues relate to patients' perceived needs for drowsiness, amnesia, analgesia, control, and specific concerns. Discussion with patients about their expectations has been shown to improve satisfaction.[8] A summary of suggested questions relating to patient choice in sedation anaesthesia is included in Box 6.4. The anaesthetist should explain to the patients that every effort will be made to meet their requests but that in some cases this cannot be guaranteed. Non-therapeutic support measures, drug dose, and selection are based on patients' requests and responses to detailed questioning.

Box 6.4 Suggested questions relating to patient choice in sedation anaesthesia

- Do you wish to be drowsy/amnesic during local anaesthetic block insertion and/or surgery?
- Do you wish to control your own sedation?
- Do you have any particular concerns relating to your sedation?
  - Lack of personal control
  - Fear of going to sleep
  - Fear of pain
  - Fear of the unknown
  - Fear of seeing the operating room
  - Fear of witnessing surgery
  - Fear of overhearing conversation relating to surgery

Intraoperative sedation must be chosen for each patient on an individual basis, depending on factors such as the nature of surgery, type of local anaesthetic block, general health and temperament of the patient and experience and aptitude of the surgeon and anaesthetist. It is important to continually focus on patient needs within the sedation triad of anxiety, analgesia, and amnesia. This will assist the choice of drug(s) and technique. A wide variety of drugs and techniques are available, ranging from simple distraction therapy through to intravenous infusion, where potential loss of consciousness and protective reflexes may occur. It is most important that the drugs and techniques used provide a margin of safety which is wide enough to render unintended loss of consciousness unlikely.

Administration of sedative drugs results in a continuum from drowsiness to deep sleep (Figure 6.3) and can progress quickly to unconsciousness or general anaesthesia. Once this has happened the sedationist has become an anaesthetist, whether or not this was intended, and the same standard of monitoring and expertise as for general anaesthetic care is required. This rate of progression may be dependent upon patient susceptibility to drugs, drug overdose, choice of drug, drug combinations, and route of administration.

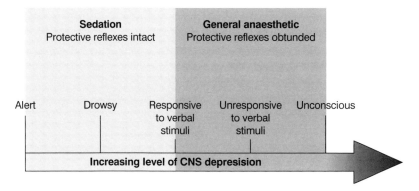

Figure 6.3 Continuum of depth of consciousness between sedation and general anaesthesia.

Safety and monitoring

Sedation often engenders an attitude of complacency and assumed safety. However, when large groups of patients are reviewed, frequent and serious complications do occur in sedated patients, mostly from ventilatory depression.[9] Anaesthetic vigilance is therefore of paramount importance. There are limitations to human performance and it is well recognised that human error is a major contributor to anaesthetic mishaps.[10] Many human errors can be forestalled by attentive monitoring and sophisticated equipment design, whereby problems are detected before they cause harm. It is essential to have an experienced sedationist, preferably an anaesthetist, to monitor and maintain safe levels of sedation. This person should not be involved in the procedure being undertaken, so that full attention is paid to patient monitoring. Patients' responses to sedative agents vary considerably. It is therefore important that the anaesthetist monitors as carefully for sedation as for general anaesthesia. Extreme care is needed when sedation is provided by non-anaesthetists and various guidelines have been produced to offer assistance in this area.[11]

The choice of monitoring should take into consideration the procedure being performed as well as any underlying medical problems that the patient may have. Essential and useful monitors for sedation are summarised in Box 6.5.

Level of consciousness
Monitoring of patients' response to verbal commands serves as a guide to their level of consciousness and is considered essential. At all times, patients must be rousable to verbal stimuli;[11] however, the sedation level will vary during the surgical procedure. It is useful to use a simple, practical scoring

133

Box 6.5 Recommended monitoring for patients receiving sedation anaesthesia

Level of consciousness:	Sedation score*
Oxygenation:	Pulse oximetry*
Ventilation:	Respiratory rate*
	Expiratory CO_2
Circulation:	Heart rate*
	Blood pressure*
	Electrocardiography

* Considered essential

system to monitor the patient's sedation level. The one I favour is a simple sedation score (Box 6.6). Other scoring systems have been used such as the Ramsay Scale,[12] the Observer's Assessment of Alertness/Sedation Scale (OAASS),[13] and the sedation visual analogue scale,[14] but all have significant limitations for clinical use.

Box 6.6 Simple sedation score

- Fully awake
- Drowsy
- Eyes closed but rousable to command
- Eyes closed but rousable to mild physical stimulation
- Eyes closed and unrousable to mild physical stimulation

Oxygenation

Continuous measurement of arterial oxygen saturation by pulse oximetry (with appropriate alarms) is essential during sedation anaesthesia. A review of 2000 anaesthetic incident reports showed that pulse oximetry detected more incidents than any other monitor.[15] In this review, Runciman *et al.* considered that the proper use of pulse oximetry would have alerted the anaesthetist in over 80% of incidents had the incident remained undetected by other means.[15] However, oxygen desaturation is a late indicator of hypoventilation and other respiratory monitors are therefore desirable.

Ventilation

Ventilatory monitoring may be accomplished by observing chest wall movement, auscultating breath sounds with a precordial stethoscope or monitoring end-tidal CO_2. Each technique has limitations in clinical practice. Patient posturing or surgical drapes can obscure visual assessment of the chest wall, while exaggerated movement of the chest wall can be seen with obstructive respiratory patterns. Precordial stethoscope auscultation can be difficult in a noisy surgical environment.

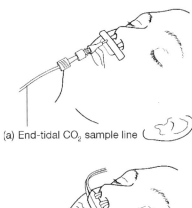

(a) End-tidal CO$_2$ sample line

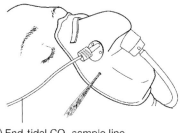

(b) End-tidal CO$_2$ sample line

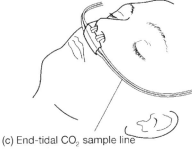

(c) End-tidal CO$_2$ sample line

Figure 6.4 A selection of commonly used systems for monitoring end-tidal CO$_2$ during sedation. The end-tidal CO$_2$ sample line may be (a) connected to a 14 gauge cannula inserted into a nasal cannula (b) attached to a Hudson mask, or (c) a commercially available nasal cannula system which has separate tubes for oxygen delivery and CO$_2$ monitoring may be used.

A capnograph which measures end-tidal CO$_2$ may detect early hypoventilation. The expired gas can be sampled through various set-ups that can be simple and inexpensive (Figure 6.4). Commonly used systems are where the end-tidal CO$_2$ sample line is attached to a Hudson mask, to a 14 gauge cannula inserted into a nasal cannula or a commercially available nasal cannula system. The latter is more expensive, with its double tubing for oxygen and end-tidal CO$_2$ sample line.

The key benefit of CO$_2$ monitoring is the continuous waveform demonstrating the respiratory pattern.[16] The shape of the waveform (Figure 6.5) can indicate normal ventilation, obstructed ventilation or apnoea. It is a

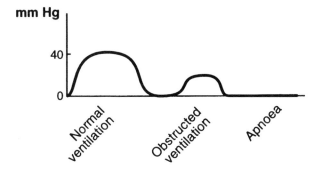

Figure 6.5 Ventilatory patterns obtained from end-tidal CO$_2$ monitoring with normal ventilation, obstructed ventilation and from an apnoeic patient.

most useful monitor in darkened rooms or where visibility of the face and chest is limited (e.g. endoscopic retrograde cholangio-pancreatography and lateral positioning).

The quantitative end-tidal CO_2 readings are less useful as they can be spurious, with reduction in measurement accuracy due to dilution by supplemental oxygen. Nevertheless, anaesthetists relate to end-tidal CO_2 monitoring, as it has become an integral part of respiratory monitoring in the anaesthetised patient and has largely replaced the use of a precordial stethoscope. Although not an essential monitor for sedation anaesthesia, this is highly recommended in high-risk patients or for procedures where patient visibility is poor.

Circulation

Blood pressure (by non-invasive means) and heart rate should be measured every five minutes. Electrocardiograph monitoring is not necessarily required in patients without cardiovascular disease. It should be used for procedures where significant fluid shifts are anticipated and in patients with significant cardiovascular disease or dysrhythmias. The sedated patient should still be able to communicate symptoms of cardiovascular disease, such as chest pain, palpitations or dyspnoea.

Oxygen supplementation

Should patients receive supplemental oxygen? Ventilatory depression precedes oxygen desaturation and when oxygen supplementation is administered, a longer lag time exists between ventilatory depression and the onset of hypoxaemia. Therefore supplemental oxygen should be administered to selected patients where hypoxaemia is anticipated, such as the elderly and those with cardiovascular disease.

Routine supplemental oxygen to sedated patients decreases patient risks but increases overall costs. It does not replace a vigilant anaesthetist constantly monitoring the patient's ventilatory pattern. Oxygen may be given *via* oxygen mask or nasal cannula. Secure taping can prevent dislodgement of a nasal cannula. A paediatric feeding tube inserted into the nares or mouth and securely taped away from the surgical field can be useful. For surgical procedures performed around the nose, oxygen tubing can be put into the patient's mouth and is tolerated particularly well. Various oxygen tubing placements can be seen in Figure 6.6.

There is concern that free-flowing oxygen, in the presence of electrosurgical coagulation, is a potential source of fire in surgery involving the head and neck.[17] Operative fires associated with electrosurgical and electrocautery units have been reported in ophthalmic and otolaryngological procedures. The use of skin preparations containing alcohol further fuels the situation if one does not allow the skin to dry adequately. In circumstances that require

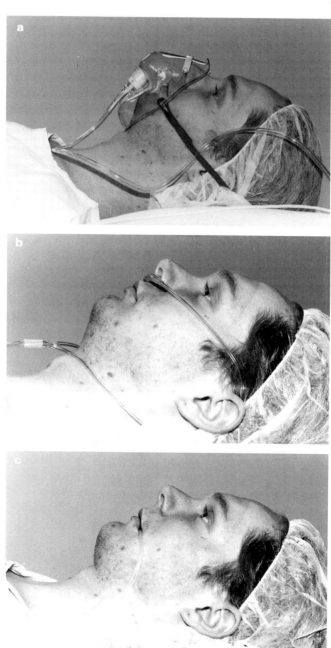

Figure 6.6 A selection of methods for providing supplemental oxygen during sedation anaesthesia. Oxygen may be provided through a clear plastic (e.g. Hudson) mask (a), from nasal cannulae (b) or from a simple catheter entering the patient's mouth (c) or nose and secured with tape.

137

oxygen supplementation and facial surgery, the delivery system needs to provide oxygen deep within the upper respiratory tract or with nasal prongs correctly fitted into the patient nares. This will prevent increased oxygen concentrations at the ignition source. Wherever feasible, all supplemental oxygen should be turned off while an electrocautery device or laser of any type is in use on an awake patient undergoing head and neck surgery.

Emergency equipment

Emergency resuscitation drugs and equipment must always be readily available when sedation anaesthesia is administered. This includes sedative drugs and pharmacologic antagonists, as well as appropriately sized equipment for maintaining a patent airway and providing positive pressure ventilation with supplemental oxygen and defibrillator (Box 6.7). Appropriate facilities and trained personnel should be available for patient resuscitation in the event of an untoward reaction. Each facility must comply with national standards, laid down by governing health bodies, to ensure safety during the administration of sedative drugs.[18-20]

Box 6.7 Emergency equipment and personnel required for sedation anaesthesia

Airway:	Suction apparatus (source and catheter)
	Oxygen with flowmeter
	Airway management equipment including facemasks and airways
	Self-inflating breathing bag valve set
	Intubating equipment: laryngoscopes, endotracheal tube (range)
	Laryngeal mask airway
Intravenous equipment:	Intravenous fluid (crystalloid)
	Intravenous cannula
	Intravenous tubing
Drugs:	Atropine
	Lidocaine (lignocaine)
	Succinylcholine (suxamethonium)
	Midazolam
	Propofol
	Antagonist drugs for narcotics and benzodiazepines
Personnel:	Registered nurse with cardiopulmonary resuscitation skills

The anaesthetic record

The sedation anaesthetic record is a communication to all staff concerned in the day surgery facility, a guidance for future administration of sedative medication and a medicolegal document. A standard anaesthetic sheet is most useful for recording sedation anaesthesia.

Key parameters to be included in the anaesthetic record include preoperative assessment details, blood pressure, pulse, oxygen saturation, and level of consciousness. The timing of drug administration, with dosages and any adverse events, should also be recorded. Minimum recording of events should be made before commencement of the procedure, after administration of anaesthetic drugs, at the completion of procedure, in the early recovery period, and prior to discharge. Ideally, documentation and monitoring of patient variables should occur every five minutes during sedation and every 30 minutes in the recovery room if the patient is stable.

Sedative agents

Propofol

Propofol has widespread acceptance as a sedative agent and is my preferred choice (Box 6.8). Propofol offers great versatility in delivery techniques due to its favourable pharmacodynamic-kinetic profile. This agent is commonly used with varied techniques: bolus dose, manual continuous infusion, target-controlled infusion, and patient-controlled sedation. Compared with midazolam, greater accuracy in drug titration can be achieved, with a reduced incidence of oversedation. There is still a risk of producing unintended anaesthesia, however, and propofol should not be administered by non-anaesthetists. Propofol can provide reliable intraoperative amnesia, but only in sedation doses.[14] If patients specifically request amnesia, 2 mg intravenous midazolam two minutes prior to propofol administration can enhance the reliability of the amnesic effect. It will also provide a smooth induction without delaying recovery.[21] Pain on injection can be minimised by selecting a large vein such as those in the antecubital fossa or by adding lidocaine (lignocaine) 1% to the propofol mixture.[22]

The cost of an anaesthetic drug is more complex than its purchase price. The direct cost of propofol must be balanced against indirect costs. Minimal turnaround time, fast tracking, reduced recovery room stay and early discharge achieved with propofol sedation will reduce overall costs incurred.[23]

Box 6.8 Advantages and disadvantages of propofol for sedation in day surgery

Advantages:	Fast onset of action
	Good intraoperative control
	Patient euphoria
	Rapid recovery
	Allows fast tracking
	Short-acting amnesic
Disadvantages:	Pain on injection
	Equipment required, e.g. infusion pump
	Cost

Recommended dose of propofol

Bolus	25–100 mg in 10 mg increments
Manual infusion	50–75 µg/kg/min
Target controlled infusion	1.0–4.0 µg/ml
Patient controlled sedation	Bolus dose: 10–18 mg.
	Lockout interval: 60–90 seconds
	(infusion rate:1200 ml/h)

Benzodiazepines

Benzodiazepines have remained popular for sedation anaesthesia because anxiolysis and amnesia are dose related and relatively controllable. Diazepam, with its long half-life (24–48 hours), has been largely replaced with midazolam, which has a shorter half-life (2–4 hours) and is water soluble, resulting in fewer venous complications such as thrombophlebitis. Midazolam also has no active metabolites, permitting rapid patient recovery. Its onset time is 2–4 minutes and as there is wide variation in patient sensitivity to midazolam, slow, careful intravenous titration to the desired clinical effect is imperative to minimise side effects from inadvertent overdosage.[24] Following midazolam sedation, patients have a slower return of psychomotor function compared to some other sedatives.[25-27]

Recommended dose of midazolam

2.0 mg if used in conjunction with propofol
2.0–7.0 mg if used alone
Infusion: 1–2 µg/kg/min

Future developments
New benzodiazepines are under development which may offer advantages over midazolam. One such drug is Ro 48–6791, a water-soluble drug which appears to be more potent and shorter lasting than midazolam. When used in combination with pethidine (meperidine) for upper or lower gastrointestinal endoscopy, Ro 48–6791 provided adequate sedation for the start of the procedure at a mean dose of 1.4 ± 0.7 mg compared to 2.6 ± 1.2 mg with midazolam.[28] The shorter duration of Ro 48–6791 was reflected in the requirement for more supplemental sedative doses during the procedure than with midazolam but, despite this, return to a fully awake state, walking unaided, and walking toe-to-heel along a straight line all occurred significantly sooner after the last sedative dose of Ro 48–6791.[28] Of some concern was a higher incidence of postprocedural dizziness in patients receiving Ro 48–6791 and the relative safety and efficacy of this new compound clearly require further evaluation before its final value can be determined.

Antagonist drugs

Flumazenil is a competitive benzodiazepine antagonist which is useful in midazolam oversedation or if immediate patient cooperation is required. It is important to recognise that resedation may occur following flumazenil, which has a half-life of approximately one hour, compared to 2–4 hours for midazolam, so caution is needed to avoid premature patient discharge.[29] Cost must also be considered, with the cost of flumazenil being approximately four times that of midazolam.

Recommended dose of flumazenil

> Intravenous increments of 0.1 mg at 30–60 second intervals
>
> Maximum dose 2 mg

Ketamine

Ketamine, a phencyclidine derivative, can be a useful addition to the anaesthetist's armamentarium for its analgesic qualities, particularly in the event of an incomplete local anaesthetic block. However, it can produce dissociative anaesthesia with restlessness, dreaming, and postoperative confusion, which can be most disturbing to the patient. This may be minimised by co-administration with other sedatives.

Recommended dose of ketamine

> Bolus dose: 20–40 mg
> Infusion rate: 5–15 µg/kg/min

Opioids

Opioids have significant side effects, including dose-related nausea and vomiting, respiratory depression, and hypotension. Sedative practices that are more frequently associated with episodes of severe hypotension are also more frequently associated with adverse outcomes.[30]

Bailey *et al.* showed that in healthy volunteers, fentanyl administered together with low doses of midazolam resulted in clinically significant ventilatory depression and hypoxaemia.[31] Therefore, care must be exercised when fentanyl and midazolam are used in combination, as their synergistic action can cause significant respiratory depression. Other opioids commonly used in sedation anaesthesia are fentanyl, alfentanil, and remifentanil.

Fentanyl

Fentanyl has an onset of action between three and five minutes and a duration of effect between 45 and 60 minutes. This is a most useful opioid to use by bolus administration and where analgesia is required in the recovery period. Small doses of 25–50 μg may cause respiratory depression when combined with sedative drugs, so vigilance and patient monitoring are important.[32]

Alfentanil
Compared to fentanyl, alfentanil is faster acting (1–2 minutes) with a duration of approximately 20 minutes. It can be administered by intermittent bolus doses or, preferably, by continuous infusion, where patients experience fewer side effects.[33]

Remifentanil
Remifentanil is a new opioid analgesic that undergoes rapid metabolism by non-specific blood and tissue esterases.[34-36] It can be administered by bolus dose or continuous infusion. Its rapid onset and elimination make it ideally suited to continuous infusion, allowing precise control of its analgesic effect and rapid recovery from its sedative and respiratory depressant effect.[37] Care should be taken to avoid oxygen desaturation when administering remifentanil by infusion. Supplemental oxygen should be provided and oxygen saturation and respiratory parameters monitored closely. Respiratory depression (defined as a respiratory rate of <8 or SpO_2 <90% for one minute) rapidly responds to a reduction in the infusion rate. The infusion should be discontinued when the final suture is in place. Remifentanil is a most useful opioid for intraoperative analgesia when postoperative analgesia is achieved with local anaesthetic.

Recommended dose of opioids

	Bolus	*Infusion rate*
Fentanyl	25–50 μg	Not applicable
Alfentanil	0.25–0.75 mg	0.5–1 μg/kg/min
Remifentanil	12.5–25 μg	0.025–0.15 μg/kg/min

Sedative drug combinations

Most anaesthetists combine several medications to achieve anxiolysis, amnesia, and analgesia. I choose a drug combination, in low dose, to exploit each drug's advantages and to avoid problems that may occur with higher drug doses. However, when ventilatory depressant drugs are combined, there may be a potentiation of the respiratory depressant effects.[38] This emphasises the importance of the anaesthetist's familiarity with the sedative and analgesic agents he or she uses as well as the need for vigilant monitoring and emergency management back-up facilities.

Sedation techniques

A wide variety of routes may be used to administer sedation anaesthesia, including oral and rectal, with transmucosal absorption by oral and nasal routes. Slow onset time and large individual variation, with unpredictability of response, limit the use of these routes in anaesthesia.

Inhalation techniques

This has been a popular technique with dental practitioners for many years, mainly using nitrous oxide. Low concentrations of this gas alleviate fear, reduce pain, and improve patient cooperation. Other inhalation agents that may be useful for sedation anaesthesia are those with high MAC values, which give a wide safety margin between sedation and general anaesthesia. Gases with low blood gas solubility will provide rapid induction and recovery. Recently, enthusiasts have used sevoflurane as a sedative agent, with the advantages of smooth sedation control and rapid recovery.[39] A nasal mask was used to deliver 3 l/min of 100% oxygen with sevoflurane added to produce an end-expired concentration of 0.8–1.5%.[39] Airway reflexes can sometimes be depressed with inhaled sedatives, depending on the concentration of the agent used. Constant vigilance is therefore required to avoid unintentional general anaesthesia.[40]

The main issue that limits inhalation sedation anaesthesia is pollution. Inhalation techniques require close-fitting nasal masks, facemasks or mouthpieces to ensure adequate drug delivery and to minimise pollution. These may be uncomfortable for the patient. Adequate scavenging is difficult, with some anaesthetic gas invariably escaping into the air. Chronic occupational exposure remains a problem for anaesthetists because of the detrimental effects that may ensue.[41] Intravenous infusion of short-acting sedative agents therefore remains the most preferable route of sedative administration.

Intravenous techniques

Propofol is widely used in adults for sedation during regional anaesthesia, endoscopic, and radiological procedures.[42] Because of its favourable pharmacokinetic and pharmacodynamic properties, propofol is the agent of choice for both manually controlled and target-controlled infusion techniques as well as for patient-controlled sedation. Midazolam in small doses (2 mg) is also regularly used as an adjunct to propofol sedation, to enhance the amnesic qualities of the technique.[21]

Manually repeated bolus injection technique
This is a commonly used technique for procedures under 30 minutes. Disadvantages include the numerous interventions required by the anaes-

thetist and wide swings in propofol blood levels resulting in abrupt changes in sedation levels and blood pressure decreases (Fig. 6.7).

Manually controlled infusion

This technique requires an infusion pump but offers more stable sedation levels (Fig. 6.7) and minimises cardiorespiratory depression.[26] Safe propofol infusion rates range between 3 and 4 mg/kg/h (50–75 µg/kg/min). Mackenzie and Grant showed that premedicated patients undergoing sedation for spinal anaesthesia required differing propofol infusion rates, depending on their age.[43] No loading dose was given and the dose ranged between 3.0 mg/kg/h for patients over 65 years and 4.1 mg/kg/h for younger patients.[43] In another study, where young, unpremedicated patients underwent extraction of wisdom teeth, a loading dose of 20 mg propofol, 0.7 µg/kg fentanyl and a propofol infusion of 3.6 mg/kg/h resulted in sedation levels no deeper than eyes closed but rousable to command.[44]

Computer-assisted target-controlled infusion (TCI)

This is a relatively new technique where the infusion rate is automatically adjusted to maintain a predicted target blood drug concentration in a stable therapeutic range (Fig. 6.7). TCI devices are computer-controlled infusion pumps. The computer program includes a mathematical model containing population pharmacokinetic parameters for the drug and infusion rate control algorithms to drive the pump. The anaesthetist selects a target blood concentration and the computer simulates the concentration profile and designs a suitable infusion regime. Hypotension, apnoea or unacceptable sedation levels are minimised by the more stable blood concentrations.

Why use TCI for sedation?

The technique is safe, effective, and easy to use with fast, predictable changes in depth of sedation. Drug-related haemodynamic and respiratory side effects from propofol overdosing are minimised. There are fewer anaesthetist interventions than from intermittent bolus injections.[45] Studies have also shown that anaesthetists feel more confident using this technique than manual infusion techniques.[46]

Disadvantages of TCI

A specific TCI device with prefilled propofol syringes can only be used for this technique. There is significant wastage of propofol for short procedures using 50 ml syringes. Nevertheless, I find this a very suitable technique for procedures longer than 45 minutes. Further studies are required to determine the cost/benefit ratio of this technique.

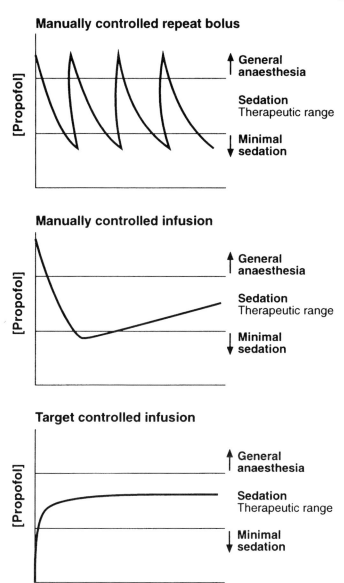

Figure 6.7 Trends in propofol blood concentrations during sedation anaesthesia produced by different drug administration regimens. With repeated bolus doses (a), concentrations fluctuate widely and may result in both inadequate and excessive sedation. With a manual infusion (b), blood levels are more constant but some fluctuation is likely unless the anaesthetist is extremely skilled in adjusting the infusion rate. With a target-controlled infusion (c) a computer-controlled infusion pump maintains reasonably stable blood levels (although variations may still occur in some patients).

145

Stepwise guidelines to using TCI for sedation

- Secure a reliable intravenous cannula.
- Pretreat with intravenous midazolam 1–2 mg.
- *Analgesia supplementation:* aliquots of intermittent alfentanil 0.25 mg or fentanyl 25 µg up to 1 mg and 100 µg, respectively.
- *Induction of sedation anaesthesia:* enter patient's age and weight into TCI device.
  Select and input target concentration:[47]

Young healthy patients:	2–2.5 µg/ml
Old, sicker patients:	1.2–1.8 µg/ml

  OR
  Stepped target concentration (for slower infusion)

Commencement rate:	0.4 µg/ml

  Increase by 0.2 µg/ml every 2 minutes.
- *Maintenance of sedation anaesthesia:* observe the patients response and alter the target blood concentration against clinical signs of sedation depth.

Choose a target blood concentration appropriate for patient fitness and the surgical procedure. For example, higher levels of sedation may be required during uncomfortable endoscopic procedures compared with lower levels where excellent regional or local anaesthesia has been achieved.

Patient-controlled sedation (PCS)

Optimum patient sedation levels may be difficult to achieve due to individual patient response to drugs, differing patient requests and varying surgical stimulation, such as peritoneal traction. PCS is an intraoperative sedation technique where patients under the supervision of an anaesthetist can administer intravenous sedatives to themselves as required. This enables them to achieve a level of sedation that meets their individual requirements. My clinical experience has shown that, given the choice, only 10% of patients prefer not to be in control of their own sedation.

Loading dose, bolus dose, and lockout intervals are programmed into a patient-demand pump by the anaesthetist. These will vary (Table 6.1) depending on the patient's age and fitness.[48] Published reports to date have shown PCS to be a safe technique with high patient satisfaction.[49–52]

Although propofol,[49–52] alfentanil,[53] and midazolam,[54] have been used with PCS, propofol has been shown to be the drug of choice, with high patient satisfaction and improved postoperative recovery. The safety and effectiveness of PCS are influenced by the sedative drug used and the settings of the patient-demand variables. Investigators have reported a stronger patient preference for patient-controlled propofol than propofol by continuous infusion.[44]

146

Table 6.1 Suggested patient-controlled sedation variables according to patient age using an infusion pump delivering propofol at 1200 ml/h.[48]

Age (years)	Bolus dose of propofol (mg)	Lockout interval (seconds)
15–39	18	60
40–49	15	70
50–59	12	80
60 or greater	10	90

Advantages of PCS
- Patients titrate the dose they require
- Patients have control of their sedation
- High patient satisfaction
- Safe technique

Limitations of PCS
- Not suitable for brief procedures
- 10% of patients prefer not to be in control
- PCS pump with high infusion rates may be difficult to acquire

Recovery and discharge

All the standards for monitoring, staffing, recovery facilities, and discharge criteria are the same as for general anaesthesia but patients may satisfy these criteria faster with sedation drugs and techniques. All patients receiving sedation anaesthesia should be monitored half-hourly until discharge criteria are met. The level of consciousness and vital signs should be recorded at regular intervals during recovery. A registered nurse should be in attendance until discharge criteria are fulfilled.

Fast tracking

If patients are alert and have stable vital signs, it is appropriate that they be transferred from the operating or procedure room directly to the second-stage recovery room (fast tracking; see Chapter 8). There are potential cost advantages with this approach, with reduction in recovery room stay and less nursing care. In a multicentre study conducted to evaluate the ability of patients to meet a standardised set of discharge criteria to bypass first-stage recovery, results showed that over 80% of patients receiving sedation anaesthesia were successfully able to bypass first-stage recovery.[55]

Discharge

Patients who have undergone sedation anaesthesia should be encouraged to walk to the bathroom as soon as they feel able. They may then be fit for discharge (Box 6.9).

147

Box 6.9 Suitable discharge criteria for sedated patients

- Stable vital signs
- Tolerate oral fluids
- Minimal nausea and vomiting
- Walk unaided
- Minimal pain
- Minimal wound discharge

Care must be taken in discharging patients who have received reversal agents (naloxone, flumazenil) to ensure that they do not become resedated after reversal effects have worn off. In this instance, sufficient time (up to two hours) should have elapsed following the last administration of a reversal agent.

Generally, sedated patients have a short recovery room time, being more dependent on the availability of patient escort, discharge medications, and postoperative appointment scheduling than on residual drug effects. Therefore these potential sources of delay should be organised in advance. The patient must be transferred into the care of a responsible adult to whom written and verbal instructions should be given. This is important as, although the patient may appear alert, amnesic drugs such as midazolam may prevent patients from remembering instructions at discharge.[56] Written instructions should also include the prohibition of driving and the operation of machinery until the day following the administration of sedative drugs.

New initiatives in sedation

Bispectral index monitoring

The Bispectral Index (BIS) is a processed EEG parameter that was specifically developed to measure patient response during the administration of anaesthetics and sedatives. BIS monitoring requires the acquisition of a special monitor and the use of a self-adhesive disposable sensor which attaches to the patient's forehead (Figure 6.8).

BIS is displayed as a single value, or a trend, on the commercially available monitor. As the level of hypnosis is increased, the BIS value decreases. Typical BIS values from my clinical experience of sedated patients are shown in Table 6.2. It should be noted that significant interindividual variation occurs.

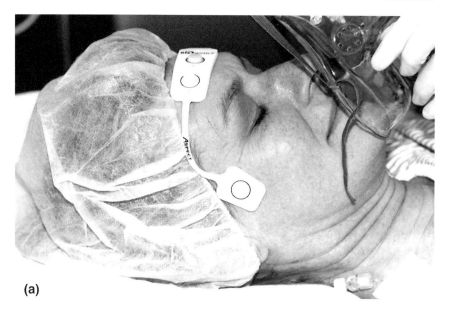

(a)

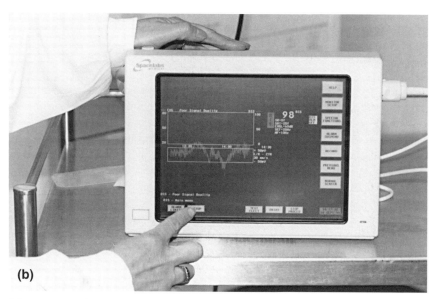

(b)

Figure 6.8 Bispectral index (BIS) is measured from a disposable electrode attached to the patient's forehead and temple (a). The signal is processed by a dedicated monitor (b), which displays the numerical BIS value (centre right) and may also display the unprocessed EEG signal and/or the trend in BIS over time, depending on the particular monitor used. Most monitors alert the user to the presence of electrical interference or other causes of poor signal quality (lower left), which may affect the accuracy of the BIS value.

149

Table 6.2 Typical BIS values for varying sedation depth

Sedation level	Typical BIS range
1 Fully awake	100
2 Drowsy	90–100
3 Eyes closed but rousable to command	80–90
4 Eyes closed but rousable to mild physical stimulation	70–80
5 Eyes closed and unrousable to mild physical stimulation	<70

BIS may become a useful clinical monitor, allowing the depth of sedation to be more accurately measured. It has already been shown to be a useful sedation monitor during surgical procedures performed under regional anaesthesia.[57] It correlates well with the level of patient responsiveness, with excellent prediction of loss of consciousness.[58] The BIS value at the end of anaesthesia has also been shown to correlate well with the time to fast-track eligibility.[59] By titrating sedation depth with BIS monitoring, patients may be able to emerge more rapidly, as less anaesthetic drug is required, with potential cost advantages to the facility. However, outlay costs for the BIS monitor and the need for dedicated disposables must be entered into the cost equation. Future outcome studies will help determine the place of BIS monitoring in this cost-conscious era.

Roving sedation teams

Sedation outside the operating theatre, such as in the magnetic resonance imaging suite, requires careful patient selection, vigilant monitoring, and adherence to safety guidelines. There may be minimal staff assistance and observation of the patient may be difficult. It is imperative that trained assistance is available and that substandard levels of monitoring are not accepted. An answer to this dilemma may be the introduction of roving sedation teams, able to provide a flexible, on-demand service. The team would provide all necessary mobile equipment for safe anaesthesia, with the assurance of optimal safety and efficiency. In addition, the team can offer preanaesthetic patient assessment and adequately trained personnel for monitoring and patient recovery, to the same standard of care as in operating room management. Recent advances in patient monitoring, drugs, and techniques have made this practice possible.[60]

Patient-maintained target-controlled infusion

The combination of patient control with TCI is an interesting concept, combining the benefits of TCI with patient-controlled feedback. Researchers using this technique with propofol TCI have demonstrated high patient satisfaction with little oversedation.[61] During a study using this technique, an intravenous propofol infusion was started at a target plasma level of 1 μg/ml. The concentration was then adjusted according to patient demand. A successful demand increased the target blood propofol concentration by 0.2 μg/ml. A lockout of two minutes and a maximum permissible target concentration of 3 μg/ml were set.[61] In the absence of patient input, the target concentration was set to gradually decline. Optimal sedation was provided at median target concentrations of 0.8–0.9 μg/ml

Further studies are required to explore patient-controlled TCI. This is presently a research tool to optimise patient satisfaction with safe sedation techniques.

Cost outcome studies

Sedation anaesthesia will remain a cost-effective alternative compared to general anaesthesia providing there is quality patient care with minimal postoperative problems. However, the problem remains of balancing patient benefits and costs.[62] We should be cognisant of the need to provide optimal patient comfort and not withhold sedation to minimise costs. Significant gains have been realised recently with the widespread acceptance of short-acting drugs for sedation with minimal side effects and fast tracking of patients with earlier discharge. More cost outcome studies are required to identify the place of sedation anaesthesia in day surgery practice.

Summary

Most patients will experience some degree of perioperative anxiety, they will want to be at varying levels of sleepiness (from wide awake to unconscious) and may require some supplemental analgesia to cover local anaesthetic injection or more extensive surgery. These three aspects, the triad of sedation, may be provided by various "sedative" medications, titrated to effect and provided to meet the specific needs of each patient and procedure. The most commonly used medications are midazolam and propofol, with short-acting opioids added for analgesia. Combinations may enhance the sedative effect but may also increase side effects. Some inhalational drugs may also be excellent sedatives, but logistical problems in their delivery limit their usefulness.

Selection criteria, monitoring, and recovery standards should be similar to general anaesthesia but patients generally move through the system faster. Sedation may be even easier to regulate using new drugs like remifentanil and new techniques such as target-controlled infusion and BIS monitoring. Patient-controlled (or maintained) sedation may further improve acceptability and enhance safety. The use of sedation in place of general anaesthesia offers many benefits and few disadvantages and its use should be encouraged.

1   Bissonnette B, Swan H, Ravussin P, Un V. Neurolept anesthesia: current status. *Can J Anaesth* 1999;**46**:154–68.
2   Smith I. Monitored anesthesia care: how much sedation, how much analgesia? *J Clin Anesth* 1996;**8**:76S–80S.
3   Koch ME, Kain ZN, Ayoub C, Rosenbaum SH. The sedative and analgesic sparing effect of music. *Anesthesiology* 1998;**89**:300–6.
4   Kruse GD, Pearson RC. Monitored anesthesia care. In: Rogers MC, Tinker J, Covino BG, Longnecker DE, eds. *Principles and practice of anesthesiology*. St. Louis: Mosby, 1993:2325–8.
5   Chung F, Mezei G, Tong D. Adverse events in ambulatory surgery. A comparison between elderly and younger patients. *Can J Anaesth* 1999;**46**:309–21.
6   Solomon SA, Kajla VK, Banerjee AK. Can the elderly tolerate endoscopy without sedation? *J Roy Coll Physic Lond* 1994;**28**:407–10.
7   Rudkin GE. Patient choice in sedation anaesthesia and recovery room analgesia. *Amb Surg* 1994;**2**:75–80.
8   Schutz SM, Lee JG, Schmitt CM, Almon M, Baillie J. Clues to patient dissatisfaction with conscious sedation for colonoscopy. *Am J Gastroenterol* 1994;**89**:1476–9.
9   Benjamin SB. Complications of conscious sedation. *Gastrointest Endosc Clin N Am* 1996;**6**:277–86.
10 Runciman WB, Sellen A, Webb RK *et al*. The Australian Incident Monitoring Study. Errors, incidents and accidents in anaesthetic practice. *Anaesth Intens Care* 1993;**21**:506–19.
11 Royal College of Surgeons of England. *Commission on the Provision of Surgical Services. Report of the working party on guidelines for sedation by non-anaesthetists*. London: HMSO, 1993.
12 Ramsay MAE, Savege TM, Simpson BRJ, Goodwin R. Controlled sedation with alphaxalone/alphadolone. *Br Med J* 1974;**2**:656–9.
13 Chernik DA, Gillings D, Laine H *et al*. Validity and reliability of the observer's assessment of alertness/sedation scale: study with intravenous midazolam. *J Clin Psychopharm* 1990;**10**:244–51.
14 Smith I, Monk TG, White PF, Ding Y. Propofol infusion during regional anesthesia: sedative, amnestic and anxiolytic properties. *Anesth Analg* 1994;**79**:313–19.
15 Runciman WB, Webb RK, Barker L, Currie M. The Australian Incident Monitoring Study. The pulse oximeter: applications and limitations–an analysis of 2000 incident reports. *Anaesth Intens Care* 1993;**21**:543–50.
16 Bennett J, Petersen T, Burleson JA. Capnography and ventilatory assessment during ambulatory dentoalveolar surgery. *J Oral Maxillofac Surg* 1997;**55**:921–5.
17 Reyes RJ, Smith AA, Mascaro JR, Windle BH. Supplemental oxygen: ensuring its safe delivery during facial surgery. *Plast Reconstr Surg* 1995;**95**:924–8.
18 Faculty of Anaesthetists, Royal Australasian College of Surgeons. *Sedation for diagnostic and minor surgical procedures*. Melbourne: Faculty of Anaesthetists, Royal Australasian College of Surgeons, 1991.
19 Association of Anaesthetists of Great Britain and Ireland. *Recommendations for standards of monitoring during anaesthesia and recovery*, revised edition. London: AAGBI 1994.
20 American Society of Anesthesiologists. Standards for basic intraoperative monitoring. In: *ASA Directory of Members*. Park Ridge, Ill: ASA, 1994:735.
21 Taylor E, Ghouri AF, White PF. Midazolam in combination with propofol for sedation during local anesthesia. *J Clin Anesth* 1992;**4**:213–16.
22 King SY, Davis FM, Wells JE, Murchison DJ, Pryor PJ. Lidocaine for the prevention of pain due to injection of propofol. *Anesth Analg* 1992;**74**:246–9.
23 Hitchcock M, Rudkin G. The real cost of total intravenous anaesthesia: cost versus price. *Amb Surg* 1995;**3**:43–8.
24 Richards A, Griffiths M, Scully C. Wide variation in patient response to midazolam sedation for outpatient oral surgery. *Oral Surg Oral Med Oral Path* 1993;**76**:408–11.

25 White PF, Negus JB. Sedative infusions during local and regional anesthesia: a comparison of midazolam and propofol. *J Clin Anesth* 1991;**3**:32–9.

26 Urquhart ML, White PF. Comparison of sedative infusions during regional anesthesia–methohexital, etomidate and midazolam. *Anesth Analg* 1989;**68**:249–54.

27 Hegarty JE, Dundee JW. Sequelae after the intravenous injection of three benzodiazepines–diazepam, lorazepam, and flunitrazepam. *Br Med J* 1977;**2**:1384–5.

28 Tang J, Wang B, White PF, Gold M, Gold J. Comparison of the sedation and recovery profiles of Ro 48–6791, a new benzodiazepine, and midazolam in combination with meperidine for outpatient endoscopic procedures. *Anesth Analg* 1999;**89**:893–8.

29 Philip BK, Simpson TH, Hauch MA, Mallampati SR. Flumazenil reverses sedation after midazolam-induced general anesthesia in ambulatory surgery patients. *Anesth Analg* 1990;**71**:371–6.

30 Daneshmend TK, Bell GD, Logan RF. Sedation for upper gastrointestinal endoscopy: results of a nationwide survey. *Gut* 1991;**32**:12–15.

31 Bailey PL, Pace NL, Ashburn MA, Moll JWB, East KA, Stanley TH. Frequent hypoxemia and apnea after sedation with midazolam and fentanyl. *Anesthesiology* 1990;**73**:826–30.

32 Rigg JR, Goldsmith CH. Recovery of ventilatory response to carbon dioxide after thiopentone, morphine and fentanyl in man. *Can Anaesth Soc J* 1976;**23**:370–82.

33 White PF, Coe V, Shafer A, Sung M-L. Comparison of alfentanil with fentanyl for outpatient anesthesia. *Anesthesiology* 1986;**64**:99–106.

34 Egan TD, Lemmens HJM, Fiset P *et al.* The pharmacokinetics of the new short-acting opioid remifentanil (G187084B) in healthy adult male volunteers. *Anesthesiology* 1993;**79**:881–92.

35 Glass PSA, Hardman D, Kamiyama Y *et al.* Preliminary pharmacokinetics and pharmacodynamics of an ultra-short-acting opioid: remifentanil (GI87084B). *Anesth Analg* 1993;**77**:1031–40.

36 Westmoreland CL, Hoke JF, Sebel PS, Hug CC, Muir KT. Pharmacokinetics of remifentanil (G187084B) and its major metabolite (G190291) in patients undergoing elective inpatient surgery. *Anesthesiology* 1993;**79**:893–903.

37 Rosow C. Remifentanil: a unique opioid analgesic (editorial). *Anesthesiology* 1993;**79**:875–6.

38 Kissin I, Vinik HR, Castillo R, Bradley EL Jr. Alfentanil potentiates midazolam-induced unconsciousness in subanalgesic doses. *Anesth Analg* 1990;**71**:65–9.

39 Hartmann T, Hoerauf K, Zavrski A, Burger H, Adel S, Zimpfer M. Light to moderate sedation with sevoflurane during spinal anesthesia. *Acta Anaesthesiol Scand* 1998;**42**(suppl 112):221–2.

40 Parbrook GD, Still DM, Parbrook EO. Comparison of i.v. sedation with midazolam and inhalation sedation with isoflurane in dental outpatients. *Br J Anaesth* 1989;**63**:81–6.

41 Shaw ADS, Morgan M. Nitrous oxide: time to stop laughing? (editorial). *Anaesthesia* 1998;**53**:213–15.

42 Smith I, White PF, Nathanson M, Gouldson R. Propofol: an update on its clinical use. *Anesthesiology* 1994;**81**:1005–43.

43 Mackenzie N, Grant IS. Propofol for intravenous sedation. *Anaesthesia* 1987;**42**:3–6.

44 Osborne GA, Rudkin GE, Jarvis DA, Young IG, Barlow J, Leppard PI. Intra-operative patient-controlled sedation and patient attitude to control. A crossover comparison of patient preference for patient-controlled propofol and propofol by continuous infusion. *Anaesthesia* 1994;**49**:287–92.

45 Newson C, Joshi GP, Victory R, White PF. Comparison of propofol administration techniques for sedation during monitored anesthesia care. *Anesth Analg* 1995;**81**:486–91.

46 White PF. Intravenous anesthesia and analgesia: what is the role of target-controlled infusion? *J Clin Anesth* 1996;**8**(suppl 1):26S–8S.

47 Casati A, Fanelli G, Casaletti E, Colnaghi E, Cedrati V, Torri G. Clinical assessment of target-controlled infusion of propofol during monitored anesthesia care. *Can J Anaesth* 1999;**46**:235–9.

48 Sparks CJ, Rudkin GE, Agiomea K, Fa'arondo JR. Inguinal field block for adult inguinal hernia repair using a short-bevel needle. Description and clinical experience in Solomon Islands and an Australian teaching hospital. *Anaesth Intens Care* 1995;**23**:143–8.

49 Rudkin GE, Osborne GA, Curtis NJ. Intra-operative patient-controlled sedation. *Anaesthesia* 1991;**46**:90–2.

50   Osborne GA, Rudkin GE, Curtis NJ, Vickers D, Craker AJ. Intra-operative patient-controlled sedation. Comparison of patient-controlled propofol with anaesthetist-administered midazolam and fentanyl. *Anaesthesia* 1991;**46**:553–6.

51   Rudkin GE, Osborne GA, Finn BP, Jarvis DA, Vickers D. Intra-operative patient-controlled sedation. Comparison of patient-controlled propofol with patient-controlled midazolam. *Anaesthesia* 1992;**47**:376–81.

52   Grattidge P. Patient-controlled sedation using propofol in day surgery. *Anaesthesia* 1992;**47**:683–5.

53   Zelcer J, White PF, Chester S, Paull JD, Molnar R. Intraoperative patient–controlled analgesia: an alternative to physician administration during outpatient monitored anesthesia care. *Anesth Analg* 1992;**75**:41–4.

54   Rodrigo MRC, Tong CKA. A comparison of patient and anaesthetist controlled midazolam sedation for dental surgery. *Anaesthesia* 1994;**49**:241–4.

55   Apfelbaum JL, Grasela TH, Walawander CA, S.A.F.E. Study Team. Bypassing the PACU–a new paradigm in ambulatory surgery (abstract). *Anesthesiology* 1997;**87**:A32.

56   Philip BK. Hazards of amnesia after midazolam in ambulatory surgical patients (letter). *Anesth Analg* 1987;**66**:97–8.

57   Leslie K, Sessler DI, Schroeder M, Walters K. Propofol blood concentration and the bispectral index predict suppression of learning during propofol/epidural anesthesia in volunteers. *Anesth Analg* 1995;**81**:1269–74.

58   Glass PSA, Bloom M, Kearse L, Rosow C, Sebel P, Manberg P. Bispectral analysis measures sedation and memory effects of propofol, midazolam, isoflurane, and alfentanil in healthy volunteers. *Anesthesiology* 1997;**86**:836–47.

59   Van Vlymen JM, White PF. Fast-track concept for ambulatory anesthesia. *Curr Opin Anesthesiol* 1998;**11**:607–13.

60   Shaughnessy TE. Sedation services for the anesthesiologist. *Anesthesiol Clin N Am* 1999;**17**:355–63.

61   Irwin MG, Thompson N, Kenny GNC. Patient-maintained propofol sedation. Assessment of a target-controlled infusion system. *Anaesthesia* 1997;**52**:525–30.

62   Dexter F. Application of cost-utility and quality-adjusted life years analyses to monitored anesthesia care for sedation only. *J Clin Anesth* 1996;**8**:286–8.

7: Postoperative pain and emesis: a systematic approach

JAN JAKOBSSON

Overview

Today minor symptoms such as pain and emesis contribute substantially to the morbidity seen in association with surgery, especially in the ambulatory setting. A number of studies have showed that pain and emesis are among the most common complaints after day case surgery, cause distress to patients, delay discharge and are also some of the most common causes for unanticipated admission.[1, 2]

The physiology and pathophysiology of somatosensory pain is now fairly well understood and is extensively described in common textbooks. The aetiology and pathophysiology associated with postoperative nausea and vomiting (PONV) is more complex and also less well described. In particular, there are many factors associated with the occurrence of PONV. There is also an intriguing interaction between pain, opioid analgesia, and PONV which should be taken into account when these symptoms are discussed.[3]

The management of postoperative pain and emesis should be evidence based wherever possible. Analgesic therapy should be based on a knowledge of the physiology of pain, the natural course of the pain associated with the surgical procedure and the pharmacology of analgesics. A similar approach should be applied to PONV management. A number of metaanalyses on the effects of pain therapy, antiemetics, and anaesthetic techniques have been published during the last years. The results of these compiled analyses of large number of patients are of considerable importance. The results of smaller individual studies following very rigid protocols may not always be easily transferred to other settings, whereas the pooled results should have more common applications.

The rational approach to postoperative pain care and emesis is to use the highest quality evidence available in a systematic fashion. Strict, structured guidelines and protocols, complemented by training of key personnel, are fundamental for success.

Postoperative pain

Pathophysiology of pain

The tissue trauma resulting from surgery sensitises the peripheral nerve fibres and is transmitted via A-δ or C fibres. At the same time, nerve impulses stimulate biochemical changes, including the peripheral release of various substances, such as "algogenes", substance P, bradykinin, prostaglandins, histamine, serotonin, and leukotrienes. These are released both at the site of injury and in the surrounding tissues. This results in an inflammatory reaction and a sensitisation of nociceptors with consequent hyperalgesia.[4] The inflammation may be worsened by increased activity in postganglionic efferent neurones following activation of spinal reflexes by nociceptive afferents. This process results in a reflex-mediated acceleration of the wound reaction.

Hyperalgesia is characterised by a reduction in the pain threshold and may be separated, in theory, into "primary" and "secondary" hyperalgesia.

Primary hyperalgesia
This occurs at the site of the injury, usually the surgical site, and is a consequence of changes in the periphery which result in increases in both the area of nociceptive activation and the intensity of nociceptive activation from the primary site of injury. This process is at least partly related to release of inflammatory substances.

Secondary hyperalgesia
This process is related to central changes which produce hyperexcitation of the spinal cord to peripheral stimuli, a sort of amplification of incoming nociceptive activity.[5]

The mechanism behind pain resulting from inflammation is known to be augmented by prostaglandins, which are released by virtually all tissues following direct trauma. Prostaglandins are metabolised from their precursor, arachidonic acid, by the enzyme cyclooxygenase. Arachidonic acid is also converted to other metabolites, such as leukotrienes and thromboxane, by similar enzymatic reactions. The cyclooxygenase pathway is considered the most strongly related to the acute inflammatory reaction, while chronic inflammation may be related more to lipooxygenase activity.[6]

Our knowledge of the trauma response, pain physiology and the inborn pain-modulating systems has increased substantially during the last decades. This has produced a tremendous growth in research to find new drugs, formulations, and techniques in order to better manage somatosensory pain. Some of this work has already had clinical benefits and today great efforts are focused on the reduction, prevention, and elimination of all kinds of pain in the perioperative period.

156

Analgesic considerations for ambulatory patients

It may be that the aim of creating a rapid recovery with a minimum of cognitive interference and a state of "street fitness" has to some extent jeopardised the aggressiveness of pain therapy in ambulatory practice. It is well known that the classic opioids may cause nausea, dizziness, and fatigue, factors that are of great importance for discharge.[7] There may also be safety concerns, such as the risk of respiratory depression and, possibly, the risk of addiction with morphine-like drugs.

There is indeed a big difference between the hospital inpatient and patients that are to be sent home. Although ambulatory patients should always have a family member or other person to escort them home, they will nevertheless be without close professional medical supervision or support after discharge. During recent years, great efforts have been focused on how to achieve good-quality postoperative pain relief, by various approaches, without compromising recovery times or delaying discharge.

Assessment of postoperative pain

One of the first steps in the process of optimising pain therapy in ambulatory surgery is to adopt a method for evaluating pain and the manoeuvres used to treat it. It is important to use a method which is simple, but as objective as possible, in measuring the individual patient's perception of pain. Such a method will enable staff to evaluate the treatments instituted in order to handle and decrease the pain experienced. Pain is an individual experience which is highly variable and cannot be accurately evaluated by an observer (Figure 7.1).[8]

The visual analogue scale (VAS) is one of the most widely accepted methods to evaluate pain in the perioperative period. Not only is this a valuable research tool but it is also simple enough to be used on a day-to-day basis. The VAS comprises a line (usually 10 cm long) representing the spectrum of pain ranging from no pain at all to the worst pain imaginable. The patient places a mark along the line to correspond to their current level of pain; this mark can be measured to yield a numerical value. Several forms of VAS are available (Figure 7.2). The simplest of these is a line drawn on paper, while others involve a slide rule-like design, with a cursor which the patient moves and a scale on the reverse from which the numerical value is read. While there is some doubt as to the interchangeability of the various designs, adequate results should be obtained if the same device is used consistently.

The VAS is an instrument which measures pain intensity at the moment it is used. More importantly, it should be used to follow pain intensity over time, aiming for a decrease in pain perception. In many hospitals, pain below 2–3 out of 10 is considered to be an acceptable goal for pain therapy

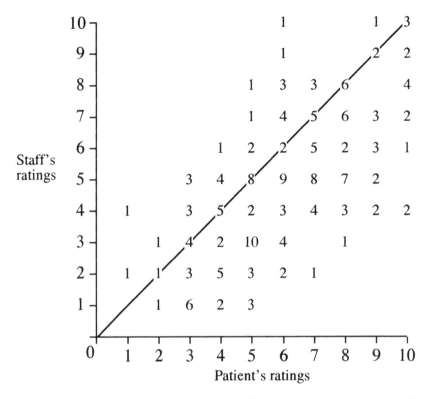

Figure 7.1 Variation in pain assessments made by patients themselves and by medical and nursing staff. 180 assessments were made; the figures indicate the number of ratings at each point. The diagonal line indicates similar pain ratings by patient and staff, numbers to the right or below the line indicate where staff underestimated pain, those to the left or above the line show that pain was overestimated. Reproduced with permission from Sjöström *et al.*[8]

and whenever pain goes above 3–4, treatment should be instituted or intensified. VAS grading should be documented; there is no reason why it should not be recorded in the same fashion as heart rate, blood pressure and other vital signs during the entire postoperative course.

Pain management

There are several options for the management of surgical pain. At the simplest level, we can administer analgesics to treat pain when it occurs. More commonly, we use various forms of drugs to work as pain prophylaxis. This requires therapy to be given before, or during, the surgical intervention, in order to reduce or prevent pain when the patients recover from anaesthesia. This is sometimes confused with the concept of preemptive

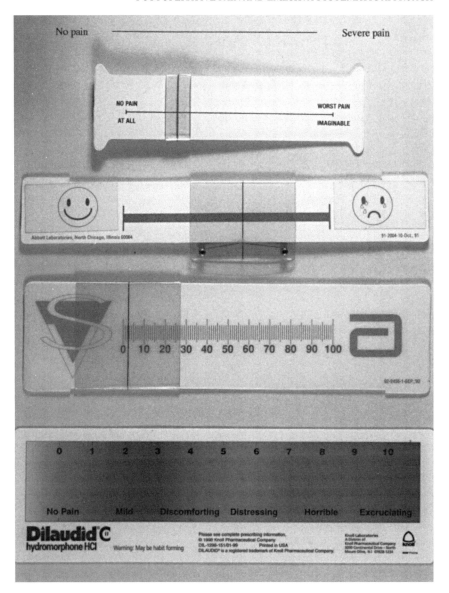

Figure 7.2 A selection of visual analogue scales (VAS) for assessing pain. The simplest involves a line drawn on paper, labelled with extremes of response and which the patient marks by drawing a vertical line. Other varieties involve a "slide rule" with a cursor which is moved along a scale labelled with descriptive terms or symbols. The level of pain can be quantified by measuring the distance along the line at which the patient makes a mark or by referring to the scale on the reverse of the ruler. Depending on the precision required, pain can be graded from 0–100 or 0–10. Verbal rating scales may also be used, where the patient assigns a number to their pain, sometimes aided by descriptive terms.

159

analgesia, for which there is some experimental data based on pain memory and the "wind-up" phenomenon.

Preemptive analgesia

Preemptive analgesia is an antinociceptive treatment that prevents the establishment of altered central processing, which theoretically can amplify postoperative pain. The altered sensory processing is caused by high-intensity noxious stimuli *via* several possible mechanisms. If therapeutic manoeuvres can prevent the sensory pathway from becoming activated from the periphery, the "insult" to the central neurones will be avoided, which should decrease the pain intensity during the postinsult period. Although there are numerous experimental studies to support the concept, the evidence for preemptive analgesia in clinical practice is today not entirely reassuring. In addition, the place for preemptive analgesia may be less important in ambulatory surgery, where minimally invasive surgical techniques may be of insufficient intensity to start a pathological pain process.[9] It is probably of greater importance to find easy and pragmatic ways to handle postoperative pain. It is of course fundamental to follow up, evaluate and, if necessary, change the pain protocol accordingly.

Prophylactic analgesia

It has become popular to initiate analgesic therapy before pain has reached great intensity or start medication in order to reach therapeutic effects by the time of recovery from anaesthesia. This is not preemptive analgesia but can be considered to be analgesic prophylaxis. This concept should be put into perspective, however. If the natural course for postoperative pain will result in the vast majority of patients having a VAS grading above 4 or 5, then prophylaxis is clearly indicated and is kinder to the patients than treating pain on request. If, however, the incidence and intensity of pain is less, prophylactic analgesia will result in more patients being treated than is absolutely necessary. For example, where a prospective randomised study shows that patients receiving prophylactic treatment have no better postoperative pain course and require no less pain treatment compared to a placebo group,[10] the value of prophylaxis is doubtful. Under such circumstances, prophylactic treatment may actually be harmful, especially with drugs carrying a potential risk for side effects.[11]

Pain therapy

In order to reach an effective strategy against postoperative pain, it is essential to have a basic knowledge of both the natural pain course of a given surgical procedure and of the drugs that can be used during this period. The literature on the natural pain course for various ambulatory surgery procedures is not extensive. There are certainly major differences in pain, which can depend on the surgeon, surgical technique and a number of other factors. It is therefore surprising that no "risk scores" have been created for postoperative pain, in contrast to PONV, where major efforts have been put into identifying numerous variables which affect its incidence and intensity.[12]

Nevertheless, looking at some typical procedures in ambulatory surgery, one may conclude that peripheral orthopaedic surgery, especially when bone has been involved, is usually associated with intense pain for several days. Arthroscopy produces mild to moderate pain for 2–3 days. Inguinal hernia repair creates continuous pain which is intensified on movement, especially walking. Laparoscopic surgery is dependent on what has been performed, cyst resection having more intense pain compared to tubal ligation, which in turn is more painful than diagnostic procedures. Hysteroscopy and dilatation and curettage produce mild, cramp-like pain for 1–2 days, while cystoscopy rarely produces postoperative pain.

Analgesics for ambulatory surgery

The analgesics to be considered in ambulatory surgery are, of course, very much the same as in all other kinds of acute pain treatment. The way in which analgesic drugs are used is probably of far greater importance than which specific drugs are chosen. Indeed, this is true throughout ambulatory surgery. It is best to choose a selection of drugs and use them in a strict and predefined manner, based on evidence and previous experience.

Morphine-like analgesics

Fentanyl, alfentanil or remifentanil are commonly used intraoperatively in low doses. While they should not routinely be administered in the postoperative period, to use an opioid when other manoeuvres to treat pain has failed (i.e. as rescue analgesia) is a natural part of acute pain management, even in ambulatory anaesthesia. The choice of drug may not be of critical importance, but the correct dose and evaluation of effect are. Use small doses given repeatedly IV (for rapid onset) and evaluate the effect after each increment.

Codeine and dextropropoxyphene are still frequently used as oral analgesics after ambulatory surgery. Dextropropoxyphene is of low potency on its own and is frequently combined with paracetamol or aspirin. Most evidence suggests that such combinations are little better than aspirin or paracetamol alone. It is also worth remembering the potential risks for adverse effects when dextropropoxyphene is combined with alcohol or taken in overdose.

Codeine or dihydrocodeine may be useful to treat moderate pain, as an alternative or to complement paracetamol and/or NSAIDs. Codeine preparations are well tolerated in most patients, although PONV, dizziness, and hallucinations sometimes occur. Prolonged administration frequently causes constipation.

Non-steroidal antiinflammatory drugs (NSAIDs)

NSAIDs have become of utmost importance in ambulatory surgery. Their efficacy has been documented in several studies and their opioid-sparing effect is well known. A recent metaanalysis[13] has shown the NSAIDs to be significantly more effective than a number of other orally administered analgesics (Figure 7.3).

A great number of NSAIDs are currently available. It is hard to give any objective advice about which to choose, as there are no systematic comparisons regarding efficacy and side effects. It is also difficult to give exact equipotent doses between the NSAIDs. It is worth remembering that these drugs work through enzyme inhibition and that their time to onset is generally in the order of 30 minutes. If used prophylactically, NSAIDs need to be given early in the procedure or preoperatively. Apart from in renal colic, the oral route is as effective as other methods of administration, if swallowing is possible.[14] Dispersable forms may be useful in patients who have difficulty with tablets. There may be some advantage in choosing a drug which is available in several formulations. Thus it can be given intravenously or rectally if the patient is nauseated or not willing to swallow in the early postoperative period and an oral formulation of the same drug can

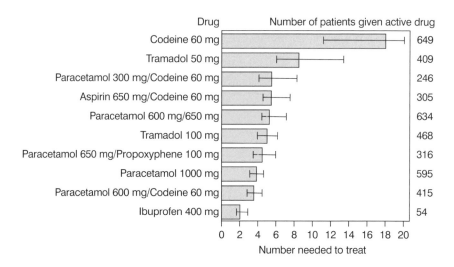

Figure 7.3 Efficacy of NSAIDs compared to alternative orally administered analgesics. Error bars indicate 95% confidence limits. Reproduced with permission from McQuay & Moore.[13]

be continued after discharge. Topical application of NSAIDs may also be effective,[15] but has not been extensively evaluated.

The NSAIDs are usually well tolerated during the 2–5 days treatment necessary after an ambulatory procedure. Nevertheless, they may cause gastric irritation, exacerbate asthma, impede thrombocyte aggregation, impair renal function and cause water retention in at-risk patients. The decision to use NSAIDs must be a balance between the specific risk factors and analgesic requirements of each individual patient. While all NSAIDs carry a risk, there is some evidence that ibuprofen and diclofenac may produce fewer adverse reactions.

NSAIDs in asthma

All NSAIDs may cause bronchospasm and worsen the symptoms of asthma. There is also a risk for "crossreaction" with acetylsalicylic acid (aspirin) sensitive patients. Fortunately, NSAIDs are widely available and used and many asthmatics will have taken these drugs in the past. Provided that their asthma was not exacerbated, there is little reason to deny these patients this valuable treatment in the perioperative period. In the absence of a past history, it is necessary to balance the requirements for effective analgesia with the risk of severe bronchospasm. Patients with mild asthma are unlikely to have their condition seriously worsened by NSAIDs but more caution may be required in patients with severe or "brittle" asthma. This approach is summarised in Figure 7.4.

Miscellaneous analgesics

Paracetamol is a useful analgesic for mild to moderate pain. It is generally well tolerated, even in patients with gastric irritation or asthma. Paracetamol probably works in the periphery, although its exact mechanism of action is unknown. Oral administration is usually adequate but suppositories are also available. Onset of action takes 40–60 minutes after oral administration.

Metamizol (dipyrone) is an analgesic that has been around for a long time in some European countries but which is unavailable in others. It has analgesic, spasmolytic and antipyretic effects. The exact mode of action is not fully described; central prostaglandin synthesis inhibition has been suggested as one mechanism for its effects. It has a well-documented analgesic efficacy, which has been compared to placebo, paracetamol, NSAIDs, and also morphine-like drugs. It is associated with relatively few direct, dose-dependent side effects, although it is thought that agranulocytosis may be a definite risk, limiting its usefulness.

Tramadol has fairly recently been introduced in much of Europe. It is a weak μ-receptor agonist and also has effects on serotonin and noradrenaline turnover, mediating analgesic effects through a reduced

163

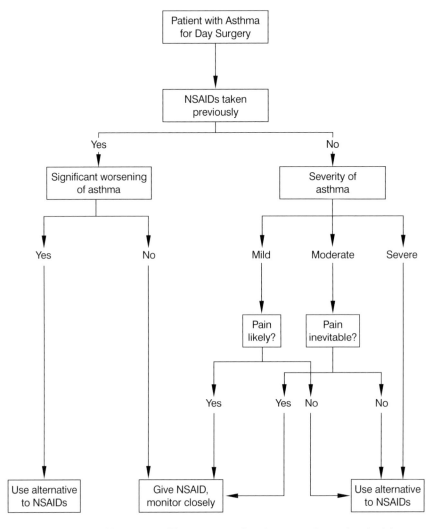

Figure 7.4 Flow diagram to illustrate a rational approach to the decision on whether or not to use NSAIDs in patients with asthma.

reabsorption of serotonin and noradrenaline within the CNS. These secondary mechanisms may be of greater importance in chronic, rather than acute, pain, however. Tramadol is available both as an injectable solution and for oral use. It has morphine-like side effects, with a potential risk for PONV and dizziness, which may limit its usefulness in ambulatory surgery. Tramadol may be a realistic alternative to morphine for treating severe pain, however.

Local anaesthesia

The use of local and regional anaesthetic techniques as an alternative to general anaesthesia is discussed elsewhere (Chapter 5). Local anaesthetic drugs also have a vital part to play in the provision of postoperative analgesia. Most procedures in which there is a skin incision or wound will benefit from the application of local anaesthesia.

Timing of local anaesthesia
Application of local anaesthesia before skin incision will reduce the intraoperative anaesthetic requirements and potentially hasten recovery. In addition, there may be a preemptive effect, although this is unlikely to be of great significance. These benefits must be balanced against the risk of haematoma formation and distortion of tissue planes which may interfere with the operation. Application of local anaesthesia at the end of surgery will still provide effective postoperative analgesia. In addition, infiltration of tissue and nerves in an open wound under direct vision is more likely to be successful than "blind" percutaneous nerve blocks.

Choice of local anaesthetic
When local anaesthetics are used for postoperative analgesia, speed of onset is relatively unimportant and duration of action is the principal concern. Until recently, bupivacaine was the logical choice, because of its long duration of action. The dose should be limited to prevent toxicity and a rule of 2 mg/kg is commonly applied. For adults weighing 50 kg or more, this will permit the use of at least 20 ml of bupivacaine 0.5%, which should be adequate for the vast majority of wounds. The 0.5% solution is preferable as it provides more profound analgesia, although the 0.25% preparation may have to be used when a larger volume injection is needed. Remember that doses of bupivacaine below the "toxic level" will still be hazardous if injected intravascularly and careful aspiration should always be performed before injection. Addition of adrenaline (epinephrine) will prolong the duration of bupivacaine, although the effect is marginal. The decision on whether or not to use adrenaline is probably better based on the requirement (if any) for local vasoconstriction.

The choice of local anaesthesia has recently been expanded by the availability of ropivacaine. Ropivacaine is similar to bupivacaine but with somewhat lower toxicity. Most evaluation of ropivacaine has focused on its use in the epidural space, where it appears to produce less profound motor block than bupivacaine. The lower toxic potential of ropivacaine should permit the subcutaneous infiltration of large volumes, extending the range of procedures for which wound infiltration is beneficial. Perhaps surprisingly, this use of ropivacaine has been largely ignored in the literature.

Site of administration

For many procedures local anaesthesia may be applied centrally (e.g. caudal epidural block), as a regional nerve block or as simple wound infiltration. The more central administration techniques offer the benefit of good analgesia with small drug doses and may be especially beneficial for extensive or bilateral surgery. In contrast, wound infiltration is extremely simple with less risk of serious complications, avoids motor and sympathetic block and, by relying on a diffuse application of local anaesthetic, avoids the risk of missing crucial nerves. Clinical experience, supported by a number of comparative trials,[16] suggests that for most day case procedures simple wound infiltration is every bit as effective as the more complex nerve blocks and should therefore be the method of choice.

Topical application of local anaesthesia may be effective provided that there is a suitable surface to facilitate absorption. Circumcision is the most obvious example and topical application of lignocaine spray or jelly provides as effective analgesia as a dorsal nerve block but with fewer complications.[17] This technique is effective in both children and adults,[18] and offers the additional advantage that topical analgesia can easily be reapplied following discharge. More recently, EMLA cream has been used for the same purpose.[19]

Intraarticular infiltration of bupivacaine may reduce pain and analgesic requirements[16] and facilitate mobilisation.[20] The addition of small doses (1–2 mg) of morphine may further improve pain relief, especially if there has been chronic inflammation.

Suggested local anaesthetic regimens for a variety of typical day case procedures are shown in Table 7.1.

Table 7.1 Suggested local anaesthetic regimens for a variety of common day case surgical procedures

Procedure	Technique
Excision / biopsy and miscellaneous skin incisions	10–20 ml bupivacaine 0.5%, depending on wound size (use 0.25% where dose exceeds 2 mg/kg)
Groin incision for varicose veins	10 ml bupivacaine, 0.5% (20 ml if bilateral)
Inguinal hernia repair	20–30 ml bupivacaine 0.5% Infiltrate around margins of mesh repair + skin
Orchidopexy	10–20 ml bupivacaine, 0.5% Consider caudal if bilateral groin and scrotal wounds
Circumcision	Lidocaine (lignocaine) jelly 2%, applied topically Reapply as needed during first 1–2 days
Arthroscopy	30 ml bupivacaine 0.5% Infiltrate portals and inject remainder into joint
Laparoscopy	10–20 ml bupivacaine, 0.5% Infiltrate portals + mesosalpynx for sterilisations

Multimodal analgesia

Multimodal or balanced analgesia is a concept of combining drugs with different mechanisms of action and/or different side effects, in order to create an additive or synergistic effect on pain perception while minimising the dose (especially for opioids) in order to minimise side effects and increase safety. Drugs which can form components of multimodal analgesia are listed in Box 7.1. It has been shown that a balanced analgesic approach combined with a strict antiemetic protocol does have a major impact on the patient's general well-being.[21, 22]

Box 7.1 Drugs and drug categories which can form components of multimodal analgesic therapy. These drugs can all be combined with local anaesthetics

Predominantly peripheral mode of action:	Paracetamol
	NSAIDs
	Metamizol
Centrally acting, oral use:	Codeine
	Dextropropoxyphene
	Tramadol
Centrally acting, systemic use:	Classic opioids

The therapeutic ladder

The concept of the therapeutic ladder (Fig. 7.5) is to start treatment with basic, safe, and well-tolerated drugs such as local anaesthetics or paracetamol. Additional analgesics are added as needed, choosing drugs which are increasingly more potent but which are also increasingly likely to produce adverse effects. The more potent drugs can be considered as "rescue agents", to be used when the basic prescribed therapy fails. These are likely to be required when the VAS is consistently above 4 or 5. When using these rescue drugs, it is wise to begin with small doses and observe their effect carefully, so as to minimise adverse effects.

Analgesia Protocol

A basic postoperative analgesia regimen which has been used to good effect by the author is the following:

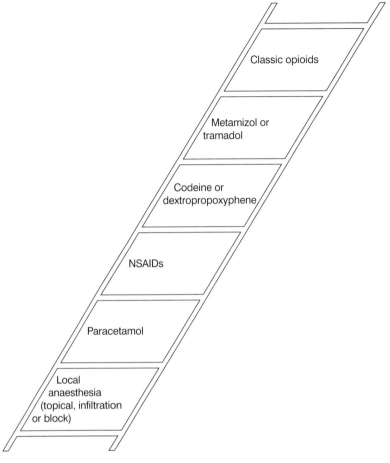

Figure 7.5 The therapeutic ladder. Treatment should commence with the treatment on the lower, left-hand step. If analgesia is still insufficient, treatment should be added with drugs on progressively higher steps.

Basic prescription
- Paracetamol 1 g
- Diclofenac 50 mg
- Codeine 60 mg

If VAS >4–5
- Tramadol 100 mg slowly IV
If VAS still >4
- Tramadol 50 mg slowly IV
If VAS still >4–5 after 15–20 minutes
- Small incremental doses of morphine 2–3 mg IV

Future developments

It is now known that cyclooxygenase (COX) exists in at least two forms. Type 1 is found at a wide range of sites (including platelets and gastric mucosa), while type 2 is inducible and associated with inflammation. Most NSAIDs inhibit both forms of the enzyme, although differences in selectivity may account for variations in side effect profiles. Selective COX-2 inhibitors (e.g. celecoxib, rofecoxib) are now available in some countries. These have primarily been investigated for the treatment of chronic arthritis. They appear to produce the usual NSAID analgesia but with fewer adverse gastric effects and no alterations of platelet function[23]. Selective COX-2 inhibitors appear effective in postoperative pain[24] but there have not yet been any comparative trials with non-selective NSAIDs. The effects of COX-2 inhibitors on asthma and renal function are currently unknown. COX-2 is found in the kidney and may be involved with autoregulation,[23] so renal dysfunction may still be possible. Current selective COX-2 inhibitors are also signigicantly more expensive than other NSAIDs. Whether these selective COX-2 inhibitors will make a major difference to pain management in ambulatory surgery remains to be seen. Their main role may be in procedures where postoperative bleeding is especially undesirable and in patients intolerant to other NSAIDs. If they do prove to have fewer adverse effects, they may also permit the use of higher doses with a possible increased effect.

There are reports that both magnesium and betamethasone have analgesic effects in some models.[25,26] Betamethasone has also been suggested to have an antiemetic action, suggesting a use in patients at high risk for PONV and postoperative pain and in whom other therapy may have adverse effects. In the author's practice, 4–8 mg betamethasone is given immediately before surgery for tonsillectomy.

Clonidine, adenosine, ketamine, and gabapentin are all drugs that have been tested in various pain situations. Whether any of these, or other adjuncts, will have a significant place in ambulatory surgery remains to be seen.

Postoperative nausea and vomiting (PONV)

The aetiology and pathophysiology associated with the distressing symptoms of nausea and vomiting are most complex. It is well known that there are a number of neurotransmitters that have an effect on the chemoreceptor trigger zone (CTZ) in the area postrema. The individual importance of each of these neurotransmitters is far from elucidated, however. There is also an influence from the vestibular system and a number of other peripheral effects may cause, or contribute to, the occurrence of emesis. For example, the gastrointestinal tract may induce nausea and vomiting by stimulation of mechanoreceptors. This information is processed through afferent pathways in the vagus nerve to the CTZ. Large amounts of 5-hydroxytrypt-amine (5-HT) are present in cells in the gastrointestinal mucosa. It has been postulated that the release of serotonin is one important factor in initiating the emetic reflex.[27]

Risk Factors for PONV

There are numerous factors associated with the occurrence of PONV. These include patient factors, surgical factors and factors related to anaesthesia and adjuvant drugs (Box 7.2).

Box 7.2 Risk factors for postoperative nausea and vomiting

Patient factors	Surgical factors	Anaesthetic factors
Female gender	Laparoscopy	Use of opioids
Non-smoker	Other gynaecological	Long duration
Age 18–45 years	surgery	surgery
One week premenstruation	Breast surgery	Etomidate
History of PONV	Otolaryngology	Ketamine
History of motion sickness	Vascular surgery	(N_2O)
	(Laparotomy)	

Patient factors
It is fairly easy to describe the high-risk patient. PONV is most likely in someone of female gender, who is non-smoking with a high body weight and aged 20–45 years. Within this group, the timing of surgery in relation to the menstrual cycle may have an impact, with the weeks immediately before menstruation carrying the highest risk.[28] Additional risk factors include a previous history of PONV and/or easily induced motion sickness.

Surgical factors
A number of surgical procedures are associated with a high risk of PONV. These include breast surgery, intraabdominal surgery and laparoscopy, ear and neck surgery. In contrast, peripheral orthopaedic surgery and cystoscopy carry a low risk of nausea.

Anaesthetic factors
While the anaesthetic technique does also have impact, this is probably less than was previously thought. Propofol anaesthesia can reduce the incidence of both nausea and vomiting, while omission of nitrous oxide (N_2O) can reduce vomiting.[29] The reduction in PONV in the early postoperative

period with propofol is quite substantial,[30] but this effect is not long-lasting. Overall, the number of cases of PONV that will be prevented by either propofol anaesthesia or omission of N_2O is probably clinically insignificant.[29]

Other drugs which can increase the incidence of PONV include the opioid analgesics. Even modest doses of fentanyl can have considerable effect, although this may often be missed as the peak effect appears to occur after hospital discharge.[31] Long-acting opioids like morphine are likely to be worse. The effect of reversal of neuromuscular block with neostigmine has also been discussed. There may be a small benefit from avoiding neostigmine, although this must be balanced against the risk of residual paralysis.[32] Combining neostigmine with atropine may result in less PONV compared with the use of glycopyrrolate.[33]

Antiemetic drugs

There are a number of drugs that are used to manage PONV. These drugs are generally antihistamines, phenothiazine derivatives or selective 5-HT_3 antagonists. Some of the more common agents are described below.

Cyclizine

Cyclizine is an antihistamine, indicated for motion sickness but sometimes used as a symptomatic treatment for opioid-induced emesis. It is a weak antiemetic but is associated with relatively few side effects. Because it is perceived as "cheap and harmless" it is quite commonly used. Nevertheless, it may contribute to postoperative drowsiness. Cyclizine has not been investigated to any great degree, although a recent study showed it to be as effective as ondansetron in reducing moderate to severe nausea after gynaecological laparoscopy.[34]

Metoclopramide

Metoclopramide is a central dopamine receptor antagonist which also stimulates gastrointestinal motility. The potential to promote gastric emptying and its low cost are often used to justify the prophylactic use of metoclopramide. However, a number of studies have shown that its antiemetic effects are little better than placebo and it is certainly less effective than droperidol or the 5-HT_3 antagonists. Poor efficacy combined with the risk of extrapyramidal side effects and sedation mean that metoclopramide is unlikely to be cost-effective in ambulatory surgery.

Droperidol

Droperidol is a butyrophenone but has properties similar to the phenothiazines. Originally a component of neurolept anaesthesia, droperidol is now used, in lower doses, as an antiemetic. The antiemetic activity is largely through antagonism at the dopamine receptor. It is associated with a number of side effects including dizziness, fatigue, sedation, and psychometric effects at higher doses.

It is difficult to advise the novice on the use of droperidol as some ambulatory anaesthetists are passionately in favour of it while others argue against its use with equal passion. The efficacy of droperidol is undisputed and some studies have shown it to be comparable to the 5-HT$_3$ antagonists in prophylaxis. This is a significant finding as the cost of droperidol is much lower than that of these newer drugs. There is much debate about the side effect profile of droperidol, however. Some practitioners feel that reducing the dose to below 1 mg (0.625 mg is commonly used) can virtually eliminate side effects while maintaining efficacy. Others point out that distressing effects such as akathisia (or restlessness) may occur even with doses of 0.5 mg.[35] It is argued that some of these late symptoms are easily missed, as they are rarely reported spontaneously and are seldom mentioned in clinical trials. Until more is known about the true incidence of adverse side effects with droperidol, it should probably not be used routinely.[36]

5-HT$_3$ antagonists

Selective antagonists of the 5-HT$_3$ receptor are effective against emesis resulting from chemotherapy, radiotherapy, and surgery. Large amounts of 5-HT are present in the gastric mucosa. Upon release (triggered by cytotoxic drugs, radiation and, perhaps, bowel handling) it binds to 5-HT$_3$ receptors on vagal afferents. 5-HT$_3$ receptors are also located in the brainstem vomiting centre.

Ondansetron was developed to combat sickness induced by cancer treatment and was subsequently found to be useful in PONV. It was initially thought to be more effective and to have fewer side effects compared to conventional treatments but this impression is changing. Ondansetron does not produce extrapyramidal reactions but other side effects do occur. Much of the evidence in support of ondansetron has compared it to placebo or metoclopramide. Dose and timing of administration are of course important, with 8 mg given towards the end of surgery appearing to be optimal. A recent metaanalysis concluded that where the risk of PONV is high (40–60% in untreated patients), for every 100 patients receiving an adequate dose of ondansetron, 20 will not vomit who would otherwise have done so.[37] The effect of ondansetron on nausea was somewhat weaker. In addition, of the same 100 patients, ondansetron would cause elevated liver function tests in three patients and a headache in a further three cases.[37] The 5-HT$_3$ antagonists are also expensive and cost has been a major factor limiting their widespread use.

More recently, ondansetron has been compared with low doses of droperidol (0.625 and 1.25 mg). These studies have found no greater efficacy with ondansetron for either nausea or vomiting in the first 24 hours after surgery.[38, 39] Even when taking into account the side effects of treatment, droperidol was shown to be far more cost-effective than ondansetron,[39] although this may change as commercial competition reduces ondansetron's cost. Combination therapy has also been shown to be more effective than treatment with a single drug. Combinations of ondansetron with droperidol[40] or a steroid[41] have shown considerably greater efficacy than ondansetron alone.

A number of other 5-HT$_3$ antagonists have been developed for cancer-related emesis and are finding their way into the management of PONV. These drugs include tropisetron, granisetron, and dolasetron. At present, comparative trials with ondansetron are largely absent. Results comparing these drugs against placebo suggest they will not be significantly more effective than ondansetron. As 5-HT$_3$ antagonists have weak effects on a variety of receptors, it is possible that slight variations in receptor-blocking profile may produce differences in side effects. Whether there are any differences of clinical importance remains to be shown in clinical studies. The wider choice of 5-HT$_3$ antagonists is likely to promote competition and ultimately reduce the cost of these drugs, however.

Treatment *versus* prophylaxis

During recent years, most studies have focused on the prevention of PONV. This is a desirable aim and represents a humane approach. In patients who are themselves at high risk or who are undergoing high-risk surgery, the prophylactic use of antiemetic therapy is both worthwhile and cost-effective. Where the risks of PONV are lower, the generalised use of prophylaxis seems more difficult to justify. Not only will liberal use of antiemetics increase monetary cost unnecessarily but there is also the cost of side effects to consider. In addition, because no antiemetic regimen is 100% effective, some patients may have drug-induced effects *added* to the symptoms of nausea and vomiting.

It is important to develop an anaesthetic technique which is associated with a low incidence of PONV and to work out regimes throughout the perioperative period that reduce the risk for these symptoms. This approach will reduce the requirements for antiemetic drugs. Because patient populations and surgical procedures vary considerably, practitioners are advised to audit their own results and adapt their personal technique(s) until acceptable results are achieved. Provision of effective analgesia, avoidance of unnecessary opioids and elimination of other unnecessary emetic triggers are likely to be key components. Preventing dehydration and hypotension may also be important. Finally, it is important to have adequate strategies to manage any patients that exhibit PONV in the postoperative period.

Treatment of established PONV

Effective treatment of established PONV is an important issue, both for those patients not given preventive therapy and also in situations where prophylaxis has failed.

In general, the drugs used to treat PONV are the same as those administered for its prevention, with metoclopramide, droperidol, prochlorperazine, and ondansetron being the most common. In evaluating the effectiveness of treatment, the natural history of PONV must be considered. Many patients experience nausea in the immediate recovery period and/or vomit once, followed by spontaneous recovery. If antiemetics are given for these early symptoms, clinical improvement may often be falsely attributed to treatment.

Metoclopramide has limited effect in the postoperative period, although it appears better than placebo.[42] Both ondansetron and droperidol are significantly more effective than metoclopramide but neither drug is obviously better than the other.[42, 43] Success rates as high as 60–70% may be achieved when established PONV is treated with ondansetron 8 mg or droperidol 1.25 mg,[42, 43] and treatment with these drugs appears no less effective than their use for prophylaxis. There is, however, relatively little data available on the comparative efficacy of various treatments for PONV.[44]

Strategies for PONV

It seems obvious that there should be protocols for the management of PONV, just as there are for pain. There seems to be less agreement in the area of PONV, however, perhaps because so many factors are involved. Any strategy which is adopted should be carefully evaluated to take into account the local factors, including individual patients, type of surgery, and anaesthetic technique. By considering patient and surgical factors, every patient can be assigned a risk for developing PONV as a guide to management. As an example, the author has found the following approach useful.

High to very high risk for PONV
In these patients, an anaesthetic technique based on propofol combined with "aggressive" antiemetic use seems to be indicated and will probably be cost-effective. All unnecessary emetic drugs are eliminated if at all possible. Prophylactic antiemetics should be given, possibly in combination; for example, cyclizine orally before surgery, droperidol 0.5 mg at induction and ondansetron 4–8 mg or granisetron 2–3 mg at the end of surgery.

Moderate risk for PONV
All drugs with an emetic potential are omitted where possible. Antiemetic prophylaxis may be required, especially when emetic drugs cannot be avoided. Possible options include cyclizine orally before surgery and/or

droperidol (0.5 mg) at induction. There should be a clear and structured protocol for PONV to follow during recovery.

Low risk for PONV

All drugs with an emetic potential are omitted where possible. Prophylaxis will probably not be required. There should be a clear and structured protocol for PONV to follow during recovery.

PONV protocol

- In the recovery room, assess pain using VAS and treat promptly according to pain protocol.
- Give affirmative support, avoid noise and resist moving the patient early in recovery.
- At the first complaint about nausea or sign of emesis:
    (1) check blood pressure, heart rate and oxygen saturation
        if BP or heart rate low, restore adequate circulation
    (2) if VAS >5–6, give pain therapy
    (3) if no improvement, administer metoclopramide 10 mg IV
    (4) if no improvement, administer droperidol 0.5–1 mg IV
    (5) if no improvement, administer ondansetron 4 mg (or granisetron 2–3 mg or tropisetron 5 mg)
    (6) if no improvement, administer further ondansetron 4 mg IV
    (7) if no improvement, add betamethasone 4 mg IV.

If nausea or emesis is severe or threatens discharge, steps 3 and 4 may be omitted.

When addressing the "big little problem" of PONV, one should also bear in mind the importance of adequate hydration and the complex interaction between pain, opioids, and nausea. Ephedrine has been used successfully in some situations, presumably by treating mild hypotension. Several other drugs have been claimed to be useful in the prevention or treatment of PONV. Transdermal hyoscine has received some attention but it is not particularly effective and produces an unacceptable degree of visual disturbance. Steroids have also been used against PONV with success and betamethasone or dexamethasone should be considered if "rescue" therapy is needed.

There may also be non-pharmacological measures to consider. It appears logical not to push the patient to drink or eat too early in the recovery process. Studies looking at withholding oral fluids, however, have not shown improved rates of PONV. Affirmative suggestions and acupressure at the P6 point have both been used with modest success in some studies.[45]

The future is likely to see the development of more selective 5-HT_3 antagonists, although these may not be significantly better than existing drugs. Antagonists of the neurokinin$_1$ receptor (NK_1 antagonists) are also undergoing early, placebo-controlled trials. While early results are promising, these drugs, like the 5-HT$_3$ antagonists, do not appear to stop PONV in all patients. Until an antiemetic strategy becomes available which can reliably and rapidly stop all cases of PONV, these symptoms will remain a problem in ambulatory surgery.

Summary

Postoperative pain and emesis are two of the major postoperative problems to manage in ambulatory surgical patients. There should be strict and clear guidelines that should be followed, although these need to be evaluated continuously and modified if needed. The management of pain and PONV should be two of the quality indicators for an ambulatory unit which are regularly audited and monitored.

The correct handling of these symptoms can only be achieved when the patient has been properly evaluated, looking at risk factors in the context of the scheduled surgical procedure. A pain and PONV strategy should be decided upon before the patient enters the operating theatre, with prophylaxis administered if required. The anaesthetic technique should be decided on the basis of a discussion with the patient, considering the surgical procedure and other factors of importance. This strategy should include not only the perioperative period but also the entire postoperative course. The patient should have access to appropriate oral analgesics and information about nausea before leaving the hospital.

In the increasing cost-conscious medical society, it is important also to have cost-benefit in mind. This is, however, a highly complex area where ambulatory patients are concerned. Some expensive prophylactic treatments and anaesthetic agents with a high direct cost may actually be cost-effective if an unanticipated admission can be avoided. On the other hand, liberal use of expensive drugs that do not alter outcome is a waste of valuable resources. It is therefore essential to monitor outcomes closely, audit individual treatments and adjust procedures accordingly.

Can we foresee any major developments in the management of pain and PONV in the near future? The selective COX-2 inhibitors will hopefully lead to fewer gastric side effects and may extend the population in whom NSAIDs are useful. These drugs are unlikely to have greater analgesic efficacy, however. New, longer lasting local anaesthetics or liposomal encapsulation of existing drugs may extend the period of effective analgesia provided by wound infiltration. Some interesting trials on catheters implanted in the wound may result in the development of patient-controlled local anaesthetic administration at home. These improvements may allow more extensive surgery to be considered on a day case basis. Further developments along these lines are likely to require novel analgesic drugs, which are at best still in the laboratory stage of development.

The most obvious development in treating PONV is the increasing availability of different 5-HT$_3$ antagonists. It seems overoptimistic to believe that these new compounds will significantly improve efficacy or reduce side effects. Commercial competition is likely, however, which should reduce the price of these drugs and render them more cost-effective. Other antiemetics may also be developed, such as the neurokinin$_1$ antagonists, although it is to early to judge their likely efficacy.

Currently the best option for both postoperative pain and PONV seems to be a systematic approach combined with "balanced" or "multimodal" therapies. Problems should be anticipated and prophylactic treatment given if necessary. At the same time, all therapeutic measures should be critically evaluated. Any unnecessary drugs should be eliminated, as they may be the cause of, rather than the solution to, many postoperative problems.

1 Gold BS, Kitz DS, Lecky JH, Neuhaus JM. Unanticipated admission to the hospital following ambulatory surgery. *JAMA* 1989;**262**:3008–10.
2 Carroll NV, Miederhoff P, Cox FM, Hirsch JD. Postoperative nausea and vomiting after discharge from outpatient surgery centers. *Anesth Analg* 1995;**80**:903–9.
3 Andersen R, Krohg K. Pain as a major cause of postoperative nausea. *Can Anaesth Soc J* 1976;**23**:366–9.
4 Levine JD, Coderre TJ, Basbaum AI. The peripheral nervous system and the inflammatory process. In: Dubner R, Gebhart GF, Bond MR, eds. *Proceedings of the Vth World Congress on Pain*. Amsterdam: Elsevier, 1988:33–3.
5 Raja SN, Meyer RA, Campbell JN. Peripheral mechanisms of somatic pain. *Anesthesiology* 1988;**68**:571–90.
6 Dahl JB, Kehlet H. Non-steroidal anti-inflammatory drugs: rationale for use in severe postoperative pain. *Br J Anaesth* 1991;**66**:703–12.
7 Anon. Postoperative pain relief and non-opioid analgesics. *Lancet* 1991;**337**:524–6.
8 Sjöström B, Haljamäe H, Dahlgren L-O, Lindström B. Assessment of postoperative pain: impact of clinical experience and professional role. *Acta Anaesthesiol Scand* 1997;**41**:339–44.
9 Penning J. Pre-emptive analgesia: what does it mean to the clinical anaesthetist? *Can J Anaesth* 1996;**43**:97–101.
10 Bjune K, Stubhaug A, Dodgson MS, Breivik H. Additive analgesic effect of codeine and paracetamol can be detected in strong, but not moderate, pain after Caesarean section. *Acta Anaesthesiol Scand* 1996;**40**:399–407.
11 Irwin MG, Roulson CJ, Jones RD, Cheng IK, Visram AR, Chan YM. Peri-operative administration of rectal diclofenac sodium. The effect on renal function in patients undergoing minor orthopaedic surgery. *Eur J Anaesthesiol* 1995;**12**:403–6.
12 Apfel CC, Greim CA, Haubitz I *et al*. A risk score to predict the probability of postoperative vomiting in adults. *Acta Anaesthesiol Scand* 1998;**42**:495–501.
13 McQuay H, Moore A. Treating acute pain in hospital. *Br Med J* 1997;**314**:1531–5.
14 Tramèr MR, Williams JE, Carroll D, Wiffen PJ, Moore RA, McQuay HJ. Comparing analgesic efficacy of non-steroidal anti-inflammatory drugs given by different routes in acute and chronic pain: a qualitative systematic review. *Acta Anaesthesiol Scand* 1998;**42**:71–9.
15 O'Hanlon JJ, McCleane G, Muldoon T. Preoperative application of piroxicam gel compared to a local anaesthetic field block for postoperative analgesia. *Acta Anaesthesiol Scand* 1996;**40**:715–18.
16 Dahl JB, Frederiksen HJ. Wound infiltration for operative and postoperative analgesia. *Curr Opin Anesthesiol* 1995;**8**:435–40.
17 Tree-Trakarn T, Pirayavaraporn S. Postoperative pain relief for circumcision in children: comparison among morphine, nerve block, and topical analgesia. *Anesthesiology* 1985;**62**:519–22.

18   Tree-Trakarn T, Pirayavaraporn S, Lertakyamanee J. Topical analgesia for relief of post-circumcision pain. *Anesthesiology* 1987;**67**:395–9.

19   Butler-O'Hara M, LeMoine C, Guillet R. Analgesia for neonatal circumcision: a randomized controlled trial of EMLA cream versus penile nerve block. *Pediatrics* 1998;**101**:E5.

20   Smith I, Van Hemelrijck J, White PF, Shively R. Effects of local anesthesia on recovery after outpatient arthroscopy. *Anesth Analg* 1991;**73**:536–9.

21   Eriksson H, Korttila K. Recovery profile after desflurane with or without ondansetron compared with propofol in patients undergoing outpatient gynecological laparoscopy. *Anesth Analg* 1996;**82**:533–8.

22   Michaloliakou C, Chung F, Sharma S. Preoperative multimodal analgesia facilitates recovery after ambulatory laparoscopic cholecystectomy. *Anesth Analg* 1996;**82**:44–51.

23   Hawkey CJ. COX-2 inhibitors. *Lancet* 1999;**353**:307–14

24   Ehrich EW, Dallob A, de Lepeleire I, *et al*. Characterization of rofecoxib as a cyclooxy-genase-2 isoform inhibitors and demonstration of analgesia in the dental pain model. *Clin Pharmacol Ther* 1999;**65**:336–47.

25   Aasboe V, Ræder JC, Groegaard B. Betamethasone reduces postoperative pain and nausea after ambulatory surgery. *Anesth Analg* 1998;**87**:319–23.

26   Tramèr MR, Schneider J, Marti R-A, Rifat K. Role of magnesium sulfate in postoperative analgesia. *Anesthesiology* 1996;**84**:340–7.

27   Naylor RJ, Inall FC. The physiology and pharmacology of postoperative nausea and vomiting. *Anaesthesia* 1994;**49**(suppl 1):2–5.

28   Koivuranta M, Läärä E, Snåre L, Alahuhta S. A survey of postoperative nausea and vomiting. *Anaesthesia* 1997;**52**:443–9.

29   Tramèr M, Moore A, McQuay H. Meta-analytic comparison of prophylactic antiemetic efficacy for postoperative nausea and vomiting: propofol anaesthesia *vs* omitting nitrous oxide *vs* total i.v. anaesthesia with propofol. *Br J Anaesth* 1997;**78**:256–9.

30   Tramèr M, Moore A, McQuay H. Propofol anaesthesia and postoperative nausea and vomiting: quantitative systemic review of randomized controlled studies. *Br J Anaesth* 1997;**78**:247–55.

31   Shakir AAK, Ramachandra V, Hasan MA. Day surgery postoperative nausea and vomiting at home related to peroperative fentanyl. *J One-day Surg* 1997;**6**(3):10–11.

32   Tramèr MR, Fuchs-Buder T. Omitting antagonism of neuromuscular block: effect on postoperative nausea and vomiting and risk of residual paralysis. A systematic review. *Br J Anaesth* 1999;**82**:379–86.

33   Chhibber AK, Lustik SJ, Thakur R, Francisco DR, Fickling KB. Effects of anticholin-ergics on postoperative vomiting, recovery, and hospital stay in children undergoing tonsillectomy with or without adenoidectomy. *Anesthesiology* 1999;**90**:697–700.

34   Cholwill JM, Wright W, Hobbs GJ, Curran J. Comparison of ondansetron and cyclizine for prevention of nausea and vomiting after day-case gynaecological laparoscopy. *Br J Anaesth* 1999;**83**:611–14.

35   Foster PN, Stickle BR, Laurence AS. Akathisia following low-dose droperidol for antiemesis in day-case patients. *Anaesthesia* 1996;**51**:491–4.

36   Jackson I. Droperidol–contra-indicated in day surgery? *J One-day Surg* 1999;**8**(4):14–15.

37   Tramèr MR, Reynolds JM, Moore RA, McQuay HJ. Efficacy, dose-response, and safety of ondansetron in prevention of postoperative nausea and vomiting. A quantitative systematic review of randomized placebo-controlled trials. *Anesthesiology* 1997;**87**:1277–89.

38   Fortney JT, Gan TJ, Graczyk S *et al*. A comparison of the efficacy, safety, and patient satis-faction of ondansetron versus droperidol as antiemetics for elective outpatient surgical procedures. *Anesth Analg* 1998;**86**:731–8.

39   Tang J, Watcha MF, White PF. A comparison of costs and efficacy of ondansetron and droperidol as prophylactic antiemetic therapy for elective outpatient gynecologic proce-dures. *Anesth Analg* 1996;**83**:304–13.

40   McKenzie R, Lim NT, Riley TJ, Hamilton DL. Droperidol/ondansetron combination controls nausea and vomiting after tubal banding. *Anesth Analg* 1996;**83**:1218–22.

41   McKenzie R, Tantisira B, Karambelkar DJ, Riley TJ, Abdelhady H. Comparison of ondansetron with ondansetron plus dexamethasone in the prevention of postoperative nausea and vomiting. *Anesth Analg* 1994;**79**:961–4.

42 Polati E, Verlato G, Finco G *et al*. Ondansetron versus metoclopramide in the treatment of postoperative nausea and vomiting. *Anesth Analg* 1997;**85**:395–9.

43 Heim C, Munzer T, Listyo R. [Ondansetron versus droperidol. Postoperative treatment against nausea and vomiting. Comparison of action, adverse effects and acceptance by gynecologic inpatients]. *Anaesthesist* 1994;**43**:504–9.

44 Wetchler BV. Postoperative nausea and vomiting in day-case surgery. *Br J Anaesth* 1992;**69**(suppl 1):33–9S.

45 Gieron C, Wieland B, van der Lange D, Tolksdorf W. Acupressure in the prevention of postoperative nausea and vomiting. *Anaesthesist* 1993;**42**:221–6.

8: Assessment of recovery, discharge, and late follow-up

Ian Jackson

Overview

This chapter is concerned with the care of patients after their surgery is completed. Appropriate levels of observation and monitoring of the patient at the various stages prior to discharge will be considered, as will policies for the anaesthetist leaving unconscious patients in the care of other health professionals. This will include a brief review of the legal aspects and recommendations available from various professional bodies worldwide.

Assessment of recovery will be discussed and the use of discharge criteria considered. This chapter will cover the continued management and education of the patient and their carer, the potential problems for the primary care team and the use of telephone follow-up and helpline numbers to minimise these. The techniques available for patient follow-up and audit in day surgery will also be discussed. New developments such as the "fast track" concept of bypassing first-stage recovery, the potential use of "hotel beds" and the concept of extended day surgery will also be introduced.

Introduction

The postoperative management of a patient can be considered as three stages.

(1) First-stage recovery. Initial recovery period following anaesthesia; starts from handover of the patient to the care of the recovery nurse until the patient is discharged to the ward.
(2) Second-stage recovery. Further recovery period on the ward prior to discharge.
(3) Third-stage recovery. Recovery period following discharge; continues until return of normal function.

It is important to realise that in day surgery this process requires active management and this begins with the patient's first visit to hospital. The preassessment (Chapter 1) starts the education and preparation of the patient (and in many day units their carer) for discharge following their operation.

The amount of time spent in each recovery stage varies according to the type of procedure performed and the anaesthetic technique used. Indeed, the first stage may be completely bypassed; this is the "fast track" concept which will be discussed later in the chapter. Furthermore, discharge should not stop our interest in the well-being of the patient and aftercare will also be considered.

First-stage recovery

Facilities and equipment

Each recovery bay should be fully equipped to national standards[1-3] with suitable monitoring including ECG, pulse oximetry, non invasive blood pressure (NIBP) measurement, a stethoscope, and a means of measuring body temperature. There are other pieces of equipment and facilities that need to be available within the recovery area and these are listed in Box 8.1. Some are obviously needed in each bay but most can be shared across the recovery area or with the operating theatres, depending on the size and location of the recovery area involved.

Box 8.1 Equipment and facilities needed in the recovery room

Each recovery bay:	Oxygen supply and patient delivery system Suction facilities Sharps disposal box Supply of swabs and adhesive tape Syringes, needles, and cannulae Range of oral and nasal airways Vomit bowl and tissues
Each recovery room:	Airway management and intubation drugs and equipment Defibrillator Neuromuscular function monitor (peripheral nerve stimulator) Intravenous infusion sets and fluids Cupboards for controlled and other drugs Refrigerator for drugs
Potentially shared with operating theatres:	Cricothyroid puncture set Difficult intubation equipment Malignant hyperthermia management drugs and equipment

Practical safety aspects

It is good practice to keep all cupboards containing drugs or cleaning fluids locked to ensure the safety of patients. This is particularly pertinent in the UK following poisoning incidents involving young children that have occurred on health service properties. However, this makes rapid access to these drugs by anaesthetists, members of their teams or the recovery staff impossible. We have all felt the frustration of finding that the key holder is almost invariably elsewhere in the day unit and even once they are located, finding the right key is a lottery! For cupboards containing non-controlled drugs it is possible to organise the keys to be left on a hook by the cupboard high enough to be out of reach of children. This ensures easy access to the correct key, it reduces the number of keys held by the designated key holder and they can be collected and locked away when the day unit is closed. For controlled drugs it is important to be able to find the key holder quickly. The use of a suitably bright ribbon attached to the keys with the policy that the key holder must leave this visible at all times makes their identification much easier for all concerned.

Location of the recovery unit

The recovery room or postanaesthesia care unit (PACU) needs to be situated next to the operating theatre complex. However, various designs are possible, ranging from those found in a stand-alone day unit to facilities shared with inpatient operating theatres. Each situation requires its own management guidelines. Shared facilities require considerable thought and organisation to ensure the day surgery patients receive the type of care they need. Unfortunately, a mixed recovery unit has the tendency to transfer inpatient management techniques, such as keeping patients longer than necessary and administering long-acting opioids to day case patients. This can be successfully managed but only if the problem is recognised and local guidelines agreed.

Management of the recovering patient

In the UK, guidelines from the Association of Anaesthetists make it clear that the patient remains the responsibility of the anaesthetist until they have recovered sufficiently to return to the ward.[1] The anaesthetist must ensure that the patient is left in the care of nursing staff who have been trained in recovery techniques and that they have the expertise and facilities to manage possible complications. However, it is also important to note that accountability for the patient's care transfers to the recovery staff and the nurse therefore must be satisfied with the condition of the patient and know where to find the anaesthetist should a problem arise.

Other national professional bodies, including the Australian and New Zealand College of Anaesthetists[2] and the American Society of Anesthesiologists,[3] make similar recommendations. This provides a clear starting point from which to build best practice for the management and assessment of patients in first-stage recovery. An official handover to the nurse is vital and should not be, as most of us have witnessed, a case of "dump and run". The information provided to the nurse (verbal and written) should include:

- the patient's name and the operation performed
- background to any specific problems the patient may have (e.g. deafness, hearing aids, artificial eyes or limbs)
- background of any preexisting disease or problems that may be important in the recovery period (e.g. slow pulse due to drug therapy or heart block)
- any special techniques used, use of local anaesthesia, other analgesia provided
- postoperative instructions regarding fluids, oxygen therapy, monitoring, and medications.

The anaesthetist, or in some countries a member of the anaesthesia care team, remains responsible for the discharge of the patient from the recovery area. General instructions for discharge from recovery may be used. These are best organised as a local protocol or set of guidelines, agreed by the anaesthetic department. We will consider these later in the chapter.

Monitoring in recovery

Common sense dictates that, following day surgery, not all patients will require full monitoring. The level of monitoring required will depend on the type and duration of anaesthetic used, the procedure performed and the fitness of the patient. Each patient in first-stage recovery should be continuously monitored with pulse oximetry and have their blood pressure checked during their stay.

Technology should not be allowed to replace clinical observation. It is important that the patient's colour, pulse, respiratory rate, chest movement and pattern of breathing, and movement of air with respiratory effort are monitored.

Oxygen therapy

Day units should look critically at the routine administration of oxygen following general anaesthesia. Oxygen should be administered where it is necessary or if it has been requested by the anaesthetists for a specific reason. The increasing use of total intravenous anaesthesia and the avoidance of nitrous oxide (N_2O) by many anaesthetists has removed the possibility of diffusion hypoxia occurring in recovery. Even where N_2O has been used, a period of high oxygen flow is usually delivered at the end of

183

surgery to "flush out" residual volatile anaesthetic agents and this practice should prevent hypoxia. Pulse oximetry has removed any uncertainty concerning hypoxia and recent publications support the use of oxygen therapy *only* in patients who have oxygen saturations of 92% or less.[4]

Pain assessment

One further important feature of recovery following day surgery should be the routine assessment of the level of pain experienced by the patient. Suitable scales include the verbal rating scale or the visual analogue scale (VAS). In the verbal rating scale the patient is asked to choose a word that corresponds closest to their pain. The terms *none, mild, moderate,* and *severe* are used as these seem to have the least variation in meaning between patients.[5] This is a simple system and can easily be used and recorded in first-stage recovery.

The VAS (see Chapter 7) is probably the most widely used pain assessment scale and is useful both in day-to-day assessment of acute pain and in research. This technique is less satisfactory in the first-stage recovery area, as it requires a marked degree of recovery of the patient. It is therefore more useful as part of the monitoring of the patient in second-stage recovery. Whichever scale is used, it is important to ensure that the patient is comfortable before transfer to the ward. It should be relatively easy for the anaesthetist to prescribe or administer further analgesia in the recovery area–a procedure that becomes more difficult in the ward area of most day units.

Criteria for discharge from first-stage recovery

These should be arranged locally with the anaesthetic department and be based on guidelines from our national bodies. The presence of guidelines does not remove the responsibility of the anaesthetist from this aspect of the patient's care and the anaesthetist or their deputy should agree with the decision. Typical guidelines would state that prior to transfer to the ward, the nursing staff must be satisfied that:

- The patient is conscious, can maintain a clear airway and protective reflexes are present
- breathing and oxygenation are satisfactory
- the cardiovascular system (pulse and blood pressure) is stable with no unexplained cardiac irregularity or persisting bleeding from the operative site
- adequate analgesic and antiemetic provisions are made
- there is no evidence of hypothermia or hyperthermia
- the anaesthetist is happy for the patient to be discharged on the basis of the above criteria.

A simple scoring system can be substituted for some of these criteria and several authors have experimented with such systems. One of the first of these was described by Aldrete,[6] who assigned scores according to activity, respiration, circulation, consciousness, and patient colour. Because of the subjectivity of colour, Steward proposed a simplified score,[7] which graded just three parameters (Box 8.2). With the advent of pulse oximetry, the Aldrete score was modified[8] by replacing colour with oxygen saturation (Box 8.3). These scores are commonly used across Canada and the USA, although in the UK they are mainly used for research purposes, in order to provide a common endpoint of recovery. A maximum score in both systems indicates that the patient can be safely moved from first-stage recovery but does not imply full recovery. One disadvantage of scoring systems is that they somewhat simplify the process, reducing the importance of clinical observation in our recovery staff. They also do not address some of the recovery criteria advised by our national bodies, such as analgesia, emesis, temperature, and assessment of the operative site.

Box 8.2 The Steward simplified scoring system*

		Score
Conscious level:	Awake	2
	Responds to stimuli	1
	Not responding	0
Airway:	Coughing on command or crying	2
	Maintain good airway	1
	Airway requires maintenance	0
Movement:	Moving limbs purposefully	2
	Non-purposeful movements	1
	Not moving	0

Total possible score 6
* (reproduced from Steward[7] with permission)

Once the agreed criteria (plus any special requirements from the anaesthetist or surgeon) have been met, the patient should be transferred to the ward. Again, there should be an official handover similar to that provided by the anaesthetic team. The patient then becomes the responsibility of the ward nurse until discharge.

The majority of day surgery patients are undergoing surgery that is relatively quick and have had an anaesthetic that allows rapid recovery (Chapters 2–5). It is important to realise that, unlike inpatient recovery areas, they should spend relatively little time in first-stage recovery, provided that problems with nausea and analgesia are minimised.

Box 8.3 The modified Aldrete recovery score*

		Score
Activity:	Able to move 4 extremities voluntarily or on command	2
	Able to move 2 extremities voluntarily or on command	1
	Unable to move extremities voluntarily or on command	0
Respiration:	Able to breathe deeply and cough freely	2
	Dyspnoea or limited breathing	1
	Apnoeic	0
Circulation:	BP ± 20% of preanaesthetic level	2
	BP ± 20–49% of preanaesthetic level	1
	BP ± 50% of preanaesthetic level	0
Consciousness:	Fully awake	2
	Arousable on calling	1
	Not responding	0
Oxygenation:	Able to maintain saturation >92% on room air	2
	Needs oxygen to maintain saturation >90%	1
	Saturation <90% even with oxygen	0

Total possible score 10; patients scoring ≥9 are fit for discharge from first-stage recovery
BP, blood pressure
(* reproduced from Aldrete[8] with permission)

Problems in first-stage recovery

A small number of patients will have severe postoperative nausea and vomiting (PONV) at some stage during their stay and some will experience this when they awake in recovery. It is recommended that the anaesthetic department have a standard protocol for the management of these cases (Chapter 7). These patients should be actively managed from the start of their symptoms. Severe pain can be a cause of nausea and treatment of the pain may be all that is necessary to relieve this problem.[9]

It is impossible to ensure that every patient is pain free when they wake up in recovery. It is therefore good practice to leave the intravenous cannula in situ for some time after patients have returned to the ward. This allows the anaesthetist (or a deputy) to easily administer intravenous analgesia or antiemetics should they be necessary. Fentanyl should be considered for the relief of pain at this stage as it offers ease of administration, a relatively fast onset of action (allowing quick titration to effect) and duration of action suitable to the day surgery arena. It is important to choose a suitable drug for use in these patients; fentanyl appears to offer a reduced incidence of nausea and vomiting but does require the early addition of oral analgesia when compared to morphine.[10]

The incidence of pain and PONV are two areas where the performances of individual anaesthetists can be assessed and, indeed, have a large effect on the patients' perceptions of their stay on the day unit.[11] In the UK, the advent of clinical governance may make these some of the easier standards to set and monitor. Day units should encourage their anaesthetic departments to consider this possibility.

The fast-track approach

The fast-track concept has been developed to identify those patients who do not need to enter first-stage recovery, thereby allowing savings in personnel to be made.[12] The concept arose with the observation that some patients already met the criteria for recovery room discharge upon their arrival, thereby questioning the need for them to spend any time in this area. Another aim of this system is to decrease the total length of time spent on the day unit by the patient and hence increase efficiency. There are obvious candidates for such a system already, for example patients undergoing operations by various local anaesthetic techniques (excluding epidural and spinal anaesthesia). In the USA, the use of monitored anaesthesia care (MAC)[13] provides a further group of patients who are obvious candidates for fast-track recovery.

The more modern anaesthetic agents such as propofol, sevoflurane, and desflurane may also facilitate fast-track recovery after general anaesthesia. For example, following gynaecological laparoscopy, 90% of women receiving desflurane and 75% of the women receiving sevoflurane were eligible for fast-track recovery.[14] When anaesthesia was maintained using a continuous infusion of propofol, 26% of the women recovered sufficiently rapidly to be able to bypass first-stage recovery.[14]

Criteria for fast-track recovery

The basic principle of fast-track recovery is that whenever a patient meets the local recovery room discharge criteria upon leaving the operating theatre, the first-stage recovery unit can be bypassed. As fast-track recovery is basically a North American concept, this decision is most commonly based on the modified Aldrete score (Box 8.3). More recently, White[15] has proposed a specific fast-track score, which also takes into account pain and PONV (Box 8.4). It is argued that these symptoms may be more common after general anaesthesia than following local anaesthesia or MAC.[15] Taking pain and PONV into account may prevent patients from moving inappropriately fast through the recovery process, to the detriment of their care.

The fast-track approach may have a variety of benefits. First, it would prevent day case patients who are wide awake being exposed to the "intimidating" atmosphere of the recovery room. Secondly, it would prevent congestion of the recovery room with a large number of day case patients. While these patients may not present a heavy workload for the recovery room, the logistics of patient transfer may still produce delays elsewhere in the operating theatre complex. Nevertheless, the major force driving the

Box 8.4 Criteria for fast tracking after day surgery with general anaesthesia*

		Score
Level of consciousness:	Awake and oriented	2
	Arousable with minimal stimulation	1
	Responsive only to tactile stimulation	0
Physical activity:	Able to move all extremities on command	2
	Some weakness in movement of extremities	1
	Unable to move extremities voluntarily	0
Haemodynamic stability:	BP ± 15% of baseline	2
	BP ± 30% of baseline	1
	BP ± 50% of baseline	0
Respiratory stability:	Respiratory rate 10–20 breaths/min; able to breathe deeply	2
	Tachypnoea with good cough	1
	Dyspnoeic with weak cough	0
Oxygen saturation status:	Maintains value >90% on room air	2
	Needs supplemental oxygen to maintain saturation >90%	1
	Saturation <90% with supplemental oxygen	0
Postoperative pain assessment:	No or mild discomfort	2
	Moderate-to-severe pain controlled with IV analgesics	1
	Persistent moderate-to-severe pain	0
Postoperative emetic symptoms:	No or mild nausea with no active vomiting	2
	Transient vomiting or retching, controlled with IV antiemetics	1
	Persistent moderate-to-severe nausea and vomiting	0

Total possible score 14; patients scoring ≥12 (with no score <1 in any individual category) are eligible for fast tracking
BP, blood pressure; IV, intravenous
(* reproduced from White,[15] with permission)

fast-track approach in the USA is the potential to reduce the recovery room staffing requirements and thus reduce costs. There are questions still to be answered[16] and further work is needed to demonstrate:

- the potential savings a day surgery facility may expect
- what, if any, is the additional workload for the second-stage recovery area
- what is required to ensure the safety of our patients.

There will be differences in potential savings across the world and, indeed, across different day units in the same country depending on current staffing arrangements in their first-stage recovery areas. Preliminary evidence[16, 17] suggests that these savings may be relatively modest, however.

Second-stage recovery

The patient has now completed the first stage of the recovery process but the work of the day unit and the nursing staff in particular is just beginning. Successful day surgery requires close attention to detail in all the areas covered in this book, from preassessment to the post-discharge follow-up.

The management and education of both the patient and their carer during second-stage recovery are crucial to our success. This stage more than any other can mean the difference between providing a quality service or what is merely seen as being part of a "production line" or "conveyer belt". Furthermore, success at this stage can make a large difference to the admission rate from the day unit. With this in mind, it is essential that patients are given time to recover and do not feel pressurised into leaving too early. However, it is also important that the staff have a routine for the mobilisation of patients. This routine will not only need to be different for the various specialties and operations, but also sometimes between surgeons in the same specialty and for different patients.

Environment

The use of beds is not recommended in day surgery, as they reinforce the "patient role" in the minds of our clients, their carers and even the medical and nursing staff. A further (perhaps cynical) advantage, particularly applicable in the UK, is that if there are no beds the day unit cannot be filled with overflow patients from inpatient wards. This ensures that day surgery continues in the face of any bed crisis!

Combined operating and recovery trolleys can be used during surgery and in the immediate postoperative period. The use of trolleys immediately introduces to everyone the concept that this is a short visit to hospital. Suitable trolleys help by:

- reducing manual moving of patients (reducing dangers to both patient and staff in an area of fast throughput)
- assisting the postoperative mobilisation of the patient.

Every day unit needs to evaluate the trolleys available on the market and find those that suit their patient population and the type of surgery performed. Ideally, the trolley should:

- have a reasonably thick comfortable mattress (as the patient may spend several hours on it)
- have a good range of height adjustment (a trolley that obviates the need for steps to get on and off will be inherently safer)
- meet all surgical requirements (width, height adjustment, attachments)
- meet all anaesthetic requirements (ease of tipping head down, easy to push!)
- meet safety requirements (suitable sides to prevent patient falling, able to deal with the maximum weight of patient allowed on the day unit, adaptable for paediatric use).

It is therefore obvious that anaesthetic considerations form only one part of the design of a successful day surgery trolley. Careful selection can yield benefits to all users but, unfortunately, there may also be some degree of compromise.

The day unit should also have sufficient numbers of reclining chairs to allow graduation of patients into the semirecumbent position, as this can help as part of this continual process of getting patients ready for discharge. The ward area used should also have:

- sufficient staffing to allow patient monitoring and education
- adequate oxygen and suction points or mobile equipment
- a means of monitoring blood pressure
- a quiet restful atmosphere
- privacy
- ample bathroom/toilet facilities
- a nurse call system
- facilities to provide fluids and food.

Aids to recovery

The choice of suitable food and fluids in the recovery process can make a large difference to your success rate and the quality of service perceived by your patients. Those who have worked on delivery wards in maternity units will know the effect of the smell of toast on your taste buds! It does appear to work in day surgery patients and is worth considering.

A further useful tip is the use of distraction therapy in children following their surgery. The provision of a video/television and a supply of a suitable choice of children's films and cartoons turns many screaming children (who may feel confused or sick or be in pain) into quiet docile human beings!

Postoperative problems

The major problems that occur in this phase are:

- pain
- nausea, vomiting and the inability to tolerate fluids
- haemorrhage
- somnolence
- inability to pass urine.

Pain
Pain has been dealt with in the previous chapter but there are several points that are important to this phase of recovery. First, it is important to assess the level of pain being experienced by the patient. This should be recorded in the patient's notes and there should be an agreed policy for the management of those who are experiencing uncontrolled pain. As mentioned earlier in this chapter, the VAS is more useful at this stage of the

patient's recovery. It can also be used to measure performance against an agreed standard within the day unit.

Patients may have less pain after surgery if they lie still and the use of a VAS in this situation is not sufficient. It is important that the assessment should be performed with the patient being encouraged to move the area that has been operated on. Pain level on ambulation is also a useful part of the assessment of the patient's readiness for discharge.

Medical and nursing staff should try hard not to have preconceived ideas about how painful any one particular operation may be. Only the person with pain can assess its severity. Any attempt by health professionals to modify that assessment or put it into other words is devaluing that assessment. Sadly, we have all heard comments like "Well, she's rolling around the bed and saying that the pain's terrible! But she's only had a D&C–she can't be in that much pain!". Unfortunately, this error is compounded by the fact that it is difficult for staff who don't accept patients' assessments of pain to keep it out of their faces and gestures, which does not go unnoticed by patients. This has major implications for quality of care and the patient's level of satisfaction with their management. As with most staff-patient interactions, the general approach and communication skills adopted are just as important as the specific intervention; that is, the *acceptance* of the pain, the *empathy*, and the *time* are just as important as the provision of further analgesia.

Another important point that it is often forgotten is that whatever pain management techniques have been utilised by the anaesthetist (be it the use of local anaesthetic or combinations of NSAIDs and intravenous opioids), they have a finite duration of action. Furthermore, the patient will often have been prescribed oral analgesics that differ from the drugs administered in the operating theatre. It is important, therefore, not only to provide patients with analgesics to take home but also to give them their first dose. Pharmacologically this makes sense, as it allows the analgesic effect of these drugs to build up before the local anaesthetic or intravenous opioids used in the operating theatre wear off. This is particularly true when using modern opioids with a short duration of action.[10] Attention to details such as these is required particularly when providing anaesthesia and analgesia for laparoscopic techniques such as cholecystectomy and tubal ligation.[18, 19]

We must also keep a degree of common sense when pursuing the control of postoperative pain, however. It is impossible to provide complete pain relief for all our patients and we need to avoid setting unrealistic standards that are not even attainable within the inpatient setting.

Nausea, vomiting and the inability to tolerate fluids
As stressed previously, patients with moderate or severe nausea, or those who are vomiting, should be actively managed. It is useful if the anaesthetic department and day unit have a standard protocol to follow. This ensures that each patient receives prompt, maximal treatment and that it does not

depend on the ability of the anaesthetist to leave the operating theatre and start further therapy. An example of a standardised treatment protocol is shown in Box 8.5. As patients may be unable to drink due to the feeling of nausea or their vomiting, we must ask if tolerating oral fluids should be a rigid criterion for discharge. Evidence from Canada would suggest this is not an absolute requirement.[20, 21] Indeed, aggressively pushing postoperative fluids may actually increase the incidence of PONV.[21]

Box 8.5 Example protocol for the management of postoperative nausea and vomiting

---

Group 1 Patients with mild to moderate nausea
- Patients will be given a single dose of antiemetic (e.g. cyclizine 50 mg) slowly intravenously in recovery.

Group 2 Patients with severe nausea or who are vomiting
- Give patient 1 litre of Hartmann's solution over 1 hour (unless contraindicated).
- Administer cyclizine 50 mg slowly intravenously (unless already given in recovery).
- Administer dexamethasone 8 mg slowly intravenously.

Review patient at 1 hour; if still experiencing nausea and vomiting, then administer granisetron 3 mg IV.
  Following this, patient should be reassured that all measures have been taken and asked whether they wish to go home or remain in hospital overnight. It should be explained that this is a self-limiting side effect and that no further active treatment will be possible.

Intractable PONV

The achievement of maximal therapy in each patient should not take longer than three hours. If at the end of this there is still a problem then a careful discussion with both the patient and their carer is required. Continued nausea and vomiting should not mean automatic admission to the hospital for an overnight stay. If maximal therapy has been provided, then no further active treatment will be possible and we are only offering support. The patient and their carer should be informed of this and reassured that PONV is a self-limiting condition. Therefore they should be offered the opportunity to stay in hospital but be allowed to go home if this is their wish. It is interesting that most patients prefer to get home as originally planned. I believe that most of us would prefer to cope with this problem under the care of our own families at home

Haemorrhage

Patients' wounds or dressings should be inspected during their stay in second-stage recovery. Any active bleeding should be reported to the surgeon and managed appropriately. The extension of day surgery to ENT procedures such as adenotonsillectomy and to minimally invasive surgery techniques in general surgery is increasing the chance of day units having to manage cases of acute haemorrhage. This should not present the day unit with any problems and guidelines on how to deal with the problem should be prepared. The operating theatre staff should have supplies of the appropriate sterile trays, including laparotomy sets. If the day unit is free standing and does not have on-site medical cover, then a member of the medical team should remain on-site until the patients are discharged. Protocols need to include clear instructions for the management of patients experiencing haemorrhage following discharge.

Somnolence
We should all be aware of how we can influence the recovery of our patients by the choice of anaesthetic and analgesic agents. This area has been dealt with extensively in several other chapters. However, it cannot be overstated just how important it is that we look critically at the outcomes of our individual anaesthetic techniques. Unfortunately, many surgeons can justifiably complain that procedures currently successful in the hands of one anaesthetist have a high failure rate with another. Anaesthesia needs to look at the training required for the provision of successful day surgery. Subspecialisation or a major move to protocol-led anaesthesia and analgesia are potential routes that need to be considered further.

Inability to pass urine
The discharge criteria discussed below will include a reference to the patient being able to pass urine before discharge (qualified with "where appropriate"). Once again, it is appropriate for day units to develop their own criteria, agreed with their surgical and anaesthetic staff. It would seem that there is support for discharging patients who have not passed urine if they are not in a high-risk category for actual retention.[22] Risk factors for postoperative urinary retention are listed in Box 8.6.

Box 8.6 Patients at high risk from urinary retention

- History of postoperative urinary retention
- Spinal/epidural anaesthesia
- Spinal opioids
- Pelvic or urological surgery
- Inguinal hernia surgery

Discharge criteria

Though every patient should be seen following their operation by the anaesthetist and surgeon involved in their care, assessment of when the patient is "street fit" or ready for discharge can, and should, be performed by nursing staff. Each day unit needs to identify clear discharge criteria as part of a written policy for staff to follow. These need to consider social factors as well as a medical assessment of sufficient recovery for discharge (Box 8.7).

Box 8.7 Criteria for discharge of patients from the day unit

- Vital signs stable for at least one hour
- Correct orientation as to time, place, and person
- Adequate pain control and has supply of oral analgesia
- Understands how to use oral analgesia supplied and has been given written information
- Ability to dress and walk where appropriate
- Minimal nausea, vomiting or dizziness
- Has at least taken oral fluids
- Minimal bleeding or wound drainage
- Has passed urine (if appropriate)
- Has a responsible adult to take them home
- Has agreed to have a carer at home for next 24 hours
- Written and verbal instructions given about postoperative care
- Knows when to come back for follow up (if appropriate)
- Emergency contact number supplied

An alternative approach is the use of a post anaesthesia recovery score suitably modified for day surgery. Aldrete published his modified score in 1995[8] and this is reproduced in Box 8.8. He has added five new categories to the five used to assess early recovery. A postanaesthesia discharge scoring system (PADSS) has also been developed by Chung and colleagues.[23] This uses a similar approach but does not require patients to have drunk liquids or passed urine prior to discharge (Box 8.9). Once again, these scoring systems allow a standardised discharge point that can be useful for research purposes. Whether this has advantages over a simple tick list of the criteria provided in Box 8.7 is for each individual day unit to decide. If a post anaesthesia recovery score is to be used, it is important that the scoring system is reproduced in full in the patient's care plan and that those criteria not addressed by this system are included at some stage in the assessment. While discharge scoring systems appear to facilitate rapid patient discharge, none of them has yet been independently validated.[22]

Box 8.8 Modified Aldrete postanaesthetic recovery (PAR) score for patients having ambulatory anaesthesia*

		Score
Activity:	Able to move 4 extremities voluntarily or on command	2
	Able to move 2 extremities voluntarily or on command	1
	Unable to move extremities voluntarily or on command	0
Respiration:	Able to breathe deeply and cough freely	2
	Dyspnoea or limited breathing	1
	Apnoeic	0
Circulation:	BP ± 20% of preanaesthetic level	2
	BP ± 20–49% of preanaesthetic level	1
	BP ± 50% of preanaesthetic level	0
Consciousness:	Fully awake	2
	Arousable on calling	1
	Not responding	0
Oxygenation:	Able to maintain saturation >92% on room air	2
	Needs oxygen to maintain saturation >90%	1
	Saturation <90% even with oxygen	0
Wound dressing:	Dry and clean	2
	Wet or marked but area constant	1
	Growing area of wetness	0
Pain:	Pain free	2
	Mild pain managed with oral therapy	1
	Severe pain requiring parenteral therapy	0
Ambulation:	Able to stand up and walk straight	2
	Vertigo when erect	1
	Dizziness when supine	0
Fasting, feeding:	Able to drink fluids	2
	Nauseated	1
	Nausea and vomiting	0
Urine output:	Has voided	2
	Unable to void but comfortable	1
	Unable to void and uncomfortable	0

Total possible score 20; patients scoring ≥18 are fit for discharge
BP, blood pressure
* (reproduced from Aldrete[8] with permission)

Discharge advice and protocols

It is important that each day unit has a checklist of advice that has to be supplied to the patient and their carer prior to discharge. Written leaflets given to the patient should back up all verbal advice. These should cover information about any medication and what to expect during the final recovery phase. Many questions will only occur to patients after they leave

Box 8.9 The modified postanaesthesia discharge scoring system (PADSS).*

		Score
Vital signs:	*Vital signs must be stable and consistent with age and preoperative baseline*	
	BP and pulse within 20% of preoperative baseline	2
	BP and pulse within 20–40% of preoperative baseline	1
	BP and pulse >40% from preoperative baseline	0
Activity level:	*Patient must be able to ambulate at preoperative level.*	
	Steady gait, no dizziness (or meets preoperative level)	2
	Requires assistance	1
	Unable to ambulate	0
Nausea and Vomiting:	*The patient should have minimal nausea and vomiting prior to discharge*	
	Minimal: successfully treated with oral medication	2
	Moderate: successfully treated with intramuscular medication	1
	Severe: continues after repeated treatment	0
Pain:	*The patient should have minimal or no pain prior to discharge*	
	The level of pain that the patient has should be acceptable to the patient.	
	Pain should be controllable by oral analgesics.	
	The location, type and intensity of pain should be consistent with anticipated postoperative discomfort.	
	Acceptability: yes	2
	no	0
Surgical bleeding:	*Postoperative bleeding should be consistent with expected blood loss for the procedure.*	
	Minimal: does not require dressing change	2
	Moderate: up to two dressing changes required	1
	Severe: more than three dressing changes required	0

Total possible score 10; patients scoring ≥9 are fit for discharge
BP, blood pressure
* (reproduced from Marshall & Chung[23] with permission)

the hospital and it is worthwhile for staff to provide general advice to patients about day-to-day activities such as bathing or showering, exercise, and return to work.

The difficult issue of driving must be considered and the patient advised appropriately. It is a legal requirement for patients not to drive while under the influence of *any* depressant drug and this includes general anaesthetics. There are few guidelines available in this field but those published do recommend a minimum of 24 hours for shorter simple procedures, where no opioids or benzodiazepines have been used, and 48 hours following procedures longer than two hours or where these drugs have been used.[24, 25] In the absence of more research on this topic and on the effect of modern anaesthetic agents on driving ability in the 48 hours following surgery, this would appear to be the best advice we can give our patients. It must be remembered, however, that the surgery, can also play a more major role in making the patient unfit to drive for longer periods, varicose vein surgery, inguinal and femoral hernia repair being more obvious examples.

Postdischarge

Day surgery and the primary care team

There have been many publications about the effect of day surgery on the workload of general practitioners and other members of the primary health-care team.[26–28] These provide conflicting evidence on what happens to day case patients following discharge. The picture that is emerging is that a well-run day surgery unit has little effect on the workload of GPs.[28] However, the same cannot be said of social costs to the carers of our patients. This is one area that is very difficult to quantify and it is difficult to create comparative costings with inpatient surgery, due to the large move to day surgery that has already taken place in most countries. Furthermore, as it is a cost not felt by the health service and, in most cultures, it is "what is expected by relatives" there is less chance of any major work being completed in this area.

We must consider how we would define a well-run day surgery unit. First, it is important that any day unit has a management team that meets on a regular basis with representatives of their local primary care team. These meetings should be used to discuss current problems, any planned new treatments being offered and changes to management of patients that may have an effect on community services.

The education of patients and their carers about what to expect in the postoperative period, and how to use the analgesia provided, is crucial to the success of any day unit. Simple information leaflets should back up verbal communication from anaesthetists, surgeons, and nursing staff. It is partic-ularly important to provide this information about analgesic drugs. Often in day surgery we discharge patients on a combination of tablets, for example a NSAID and a paracetamol-codeine combination drug. It is easy for patients who are just recovering from their operation to forget what they have been told about taking these tablets. Our own research has shown that up to 22% of patients reporting moderate or severe pain after day surgery are using their own simple analgesics, with a further 9% not taking anything. The instigation of an education system for patients and their carers, and the simple information leaflets described, reduced this to 2.5% and 1% respectively. Examples of two of these leaflets are shown in Figures 8.1 and 8.2.

Co-Codamol 30/500

You have been prescribed Co-codamol 30/500 for pain relief. It contains two painkillers Paracetamol and Codeine. You may well recognise that many pain-relieving drugs that you can buy from your pharmacy contain these also. However it is important that you use these tablets as they are stronger and we believe you will need these for pain relief after your operation.

How should I take it?
Usually we will have given you your first dose before you leave the day unit. When at home you should take 2 tablets every 6 hours especially for the first two days after your operation. This will help reduce the pain and discomfort you feel after your operation. After this you may not need to take these tablets so often. However it is better to reduce to 1 tablet every 6 hours at first to see.

How many can I take?
Do not take more than 2 tablets at any one time
Do not take more than 8 tablets in 24 hours

Does Co-codamol 30/500 have any side effects?
It does not normally cause any troublesome side effects. However it can sometimes make you feel sick or even make you be sick. It may also cause drowsiness or a slight giddiness and it can lead to constipation. Constipation can be relieved by eating plenty of fibre (fruits and vegetables for example). It is wise not to drive or to use machinery while you are taking these tablets. If any of these side effects become a problem then please see your doctor.

Can I take any other medicines?
Please continue to take any tablets you are normally prescribed by your GP or any you have been given by the Day Unit. However it is important not to take any other tablets or mixtures that contain Paracetamol. Please ask your doctor or pharmacist if you are uncertain.

Can I drink alcohol whilst taking these tablets?
You should not drink alcohol, as it is likely to make any drowsiness worse.

For how long should I be taking it?
You may stop taking these tablets when you feel that the pain is no longer a problem

If your pain is not relieved or eased by these tablets, please contact us.

(Produced by Pharmacy Department, York District Hospital)

Figure 8.1 Patient information sheet for co-codamol 30/500. (Courtesy of York District Hospital.)

Diclofenac

You have been prescribed diclofenac for pain relief. It contains a drug related to aspirin that is a good analgesic and also helps to settle any inflammation or swelling.

How should I take these tablets?

Take 1 tablet 3 times a day regularly for 4 days until the tablets are finished. This will help control any pain and discomfort you may feel.

What do I need to know before taking diclofenac?

Diclofenac can cause ulcer problems and so you should not take it if you have had a stomach or duodenal ulcer. You should not take diclofenac if you have had an allergic reaction or developed wheezing after taking aspirin, especially if you have asthma. Please tell us if you have had any of these problems before you take the medicine.

When should I take diclofenac?

Try to take it with food, preferably at meal times. You should not take diclofenac on an empty stomach; even a biscuit or a glass of milk is better than no food.

What if I forget to take a dose?

If you forget a dose then take a tablet as soon as you remember and then carry on with the same dosage times as before.

Does diclofenac have any side effects?

Usually diclofenac does not cause any problems but it can cause side effects in some people.

Skin troubles such as a rash or itching may occur. It can cause breathing problems such as wheezing or shortness of breath. Stomach discomfort or heartburn may also be experienced for the first time by some patients. It may cause a mild headache or dizziness.

What should I do if I experience any side effects?

You should stop taking the tablets and contact your doctor, pharmacist or ourselves, especially if the side effects persist.

Can I take other medicines?

Please continue to take any tablets you are normally prescribed by your GP or any you have been given by the Day Unit. Some medicines such as warfarin and lithium may be affected by diclofenac. Please ask us, your doctor or pharmacist if you are uncertain about how your other medications may be affected.

Can I drink alcohol whilst taking these tablets?

Alcohol may increase the chance of you having a stomach upset with diclofenac and is best avoided.

(Produced by Pharmacy Department, York District Hospital)

Figure 8.2 Patient information sheet for diclofenac. (Courtesy of York District Hospital.)

This education process should be supported by the provision of an emergency contact number that patients can ring if they develop problems. It is important to provide someone who is knowledgeable about surgery, analgesia, and the recovery process on this phone line. Each day unit needs to consider how they can provide this service within the resources they have available. Some use a rota of their more senior nursing staff, who provide cover from home utilising a mobile phone. Other day units use a hospital-based system, utilising nursing staff outside the day unit. Clear guidelines for referral either to the GP or the hospital team should be agreed, to save confusion when dealing with phone calls outside office hours.

Finally, the patient should know that they are going to be contacted by the day unit the next day to ensure their well-being. It is important to discuss this with the patient before discharge for a variety of reasons. Some patients may be staying with friends, neighbours or relations during their recovery and will therefore be away from their usual home. There may also be occasions when the patient may not want a phone call; in fact, relatives may not know they have attended for surgery. Patients have the right to say no and this should be respected. Most value the contact from the hospital, however, and many patients and their carers will save discussion of any problems they are experiencing for this follow-up call.[29] This has the useful effect of minimising the workload of both the emergency contact line and the GP.

With such aftercare procedures in place, the workload of the primary care team can be minimised in the first 24–48 hours. Despite attention to these details, up to 40% of patients still make appointments to see their GP following day surgery. The reasons for this vary and there are only some areas that we can hope to influence. For example:

- in the UK patients may visit to obtain a 'sick note' for their work
- some patients (particularly the elderly) like to pay a social visit to their GP and confirm that they have had their operation, thank them for referring them and to show them their scar!
- some patients are visiting for continued management of co-existing diseases.

Recognising this is important and needs to be discussed with the local primary care team. In reality, this may not represent an increase in workload for the GP as the patient would have attended even if they had been treated as an inpatient. However, we should still actively search for techniques to reduce the load on this sector of the health service.

Techniques for patient follow-up

We have already discussed the use of the telephone follow-up as a means of postdischarge support following day surgery. This phone call is also an ideal opportunity to gain useful data for audit and for monitoring quality standards.

Although an unstructured phone call may seem the best approach to maintain informality, a structured questionnaire should be followed when specific audit data are required. Results from our own experience of a long-term telephone follow-up[29] emphasise the value of asking about other postoperative side effects, like interrupted sleep, sore throat, headache, etc. In this study we were able to contact 77% of our patients the day following surgery. Phoning in the morning before 9 am or in the early evening after 6 pm would seem to yield the best success rate. The questionnaire used is shown in Figure 8.3.

This follow-up procedure allows constant monitoring for problems and provides early indications when a procedure is going well or badly. This is perhaps best demonstrated by an early example from our day unit. Several patients who were regular attenders at the day unit for cystoscopy under general anaesthesia started complaining of severe somnolence lasting for several days, a problem they had not experienced before. Another two patients reported severe anxiety attacks following their discharge from the day unit. Examination of these patients' records revealed that they had all received a "low dose" of droperidol (less than 1 mg) as prophylaxis against nausea and vomiting. Discussion with anaesthetic colleagues led to the removal of droperidol from the day unit and the publication of a review article questioning the use of this drug in day surgery.[30]

Other areas that we have been able to address with this information are often predictable but difficult to manage (as in persuading colleagues to change their practice) unless one has evidence of the problem. An example was the reduction in the use of suxamethonium (succinylcholine) for intubation of patients undergoing removal of wisdom teeth, as this was linked to a high incidence (40%) of muscular aches and pains.

This follow-up system only provides information about the first 24 hours following surgery. It is important for us to review not only what happens after this time but also what the patient thinks about their experience from preassessment to discharge. Due to the pioneering work of the Audit Commission in the UK, we have a useful tool for the assessment of the quality of service we are supplying to patients. The Commission asked the Health Services Research Unit of the London School of Hygiene and Tropical Medicine to develop and validate a questionnaire for patients.[31] The resulting questionnaire is extremely comprehensive, covering factors as diverse as parking, privacy, attitude of staff, and speed of recovery of normal function. This tool is worthy of consideration for use in every day unit and I recommend that if you have not used or seen this questionnaire, you find the above reference. It provides a full copy of the questionnaire and details about its development, how to use it and the results of its use in field trials in three health authorities. It is interesting (but perhaps not altogether surprising in the UK) that in this study the largest area of dissatisfaction at one week after the operation was with the facilities provided (lack of

201

Telephone Follow-up Service
Day Unit
York District Hospital

Name   Age

Date of operation   Date and time of phone call

Operation performed

Have you had any problems with any of the following?

	None	Mild	Moderate	Severe
Nausea				
Vomiting				
Headache				
Muscular Ache				
Sore throat				
Drowsiness				

How much pain have you had from your operation?

None	Mild	Moderate	Severe

Were you satisfied with the pain relief given?

Yes	No	Sometimes	Used own tablets	Did not take tablets

Has someone been looking after you since you got home?

No	Some of the time	All of the time

Did you have a problem? If yes who did you contact?

Pain	Nausea/vomiting	Faint	Bleeding	Other
No-one	GP	Day Unit	Other	

Given the choice which would you prefer for the same operation?

To have the operation and go home the same day–as this time	
To stay in hospital overnight before going home	
Don't know/unsure	

Do you have any additional comments or suggestions to improve our service?

If advice given please specify on back of this sheet

Figure 8.3 Example of telephone follow-up questionnaire. (Courtesy of York District Hospital.)

parking, lack of privacy, and lack of telephones). In fact, 47% of those with complaints mentioned these aspects of their care. Further audits and quality monitoring projects should be arranged by day units according to their patient population, type of surgery performed, and local standards.

Hotel beds

It is important to be clear about what is meant by the provision of hotel services or a patient hotel. In this discussion, I refer to the provision of accommodation in or near a hospital site that can be used by a patient following discharge from the hospital, as described by the group from Kingston Hospital.[32] Such a centre would be run by receptionist staff and would not employ nursing staff. The service would provide a bedroom suitable for patient and a carer, with *en-suite* facilities. There should be dining, kitchen, and sitting areas for the "guests" and meals should be provided. Stay in the hotel should be limited to a maximum period of somewhere between two and five days, with most day surgery patients spending a simple overnight stay.

At first, it may seem difficult to understand how such a facility may help in day surgery. However, two of the limitations in day surgery are:

- the social circumstances of the patient (lack of telephone, escort home, carer)
- medical/surgical conservatism (that is, an unwillingness to move procedures to the day surgery arena despite evidence of their success elsewhere).

Hotel beds can provide an answer to both these problems and so allow us to increase the number of patients treated on a day case basis. Evidence suggests that surgeons are encouraged to attempt larger, or different, procedures on patients as a day case if they can use hotel beds on the hospital site. They are also useful for the introduction of new, larger procedures to the day surgery arena. There are many operations, such as laparoscopic cholecystectomy, bilateral varicose vein surgery, adenoidectomy, tonsillectomy, and thyroidectomy, that are accepted as suitable for day surgery in many centres across the UK and the rest of the world. However, they are still only being introduced slowly (or not at all) in most centres. This makes no financial sense to any health service, however it is funded.

If the hotel is located on the hospital site, it offers several advantages for other patient groups. An example are elderly cataract patients who live some distance from the hospital or who have little support at home. An overnight stay in such a facility would be cheaper for the health service, than an inpatient stay and would provide a better quality of service for the patient. Furthermore, it would save the patient and the health service from having to provide a return trip the next day for an eye check. Economics once again forms the backbone of the move to the provision of hotel beds. As they are staffed purely by a small number of non-nursing personnel, they cost much less to run than an equivalent ward area.

Extending the day

This is currently a UK-based consideration and is linked to the definition of day surgery. In the UK, the day surgery model is based around a 2–6-hour stay for the patient whilst in some countries (e.g. the USA) the stay can be up to 24 hours. Protagonists of extending the day argue that changing the definition to incorporate an overnight stay would greatly increase the amount of day surgery they could perform.[33] Currently there are no published data comparing what is possible in similar patient populations undergoing similar procedures. Furthermore, there would appear to be potential overlap with hotel beds and it would be interesting to see some research done in this area. This would need to address not only the potential for each system to increase the number of patients suitable for day surgery but also the cost to the health service.

Summary

Recovery from anaesthesia may conveniently be divided into three stages. The first stage begins at the end of anaesthesia and continues until the patient is conscious, oriented, has a clear airway, and stable vital signs, and is comfortable. Patient monitoring and management are at their most intense during this early phase but modern anaesthetics may reduce the duration of first-stage recovery or even eliminate it altogether, allowing the patient to be fast-tracked direct to the second stage.

During second-stage recovery the patient is prepared for discharge from the hospital or day unit. As the effects of anaesthesia recede, problems such as pain and nausea may emerge (if they have not already presented) and other postoperative problems, such as wound haemorrhage, hypotension, and urinary retention, must also be watched for. Once patients have mobilised without problems and have received appropriate instructions and facilities for their aftercare, they may be allowed home with a suitable escort. Discharge criteria are essentially clinical in nature but may be aided by scoring systems.

After discharge, emergency support and aftercare must be available but patients should also be followed up to detect recurring, preventable problems and to audit performance. Such aftercare is especially important when extending the selection criteria for day surgery. Further measures, such as hotel beds or extended day surgery, may also allow more patients to benefit from the day case experience.

1   Association of Anaesthetists of Great Britain and Ireland. *Immediate postanaesthetic recovery*. London: AAGBI, 1993.

2   Australian and New Zealand College of Anaesthetists. *Guidelines for the care of patients recovering from anaesthesia*. Melborne: ANZCA, 1995.

3   American Society of Anesthesiologists. *Standards for postanesthesia care*. Park Ridge, Illinois: ASA, 1994.

4   Gift AG, Stanik J, Karpenick J, Whitmore K, Bolgiano CS. Oxygen saturation in postoperative patients at low risk for hypoxemia: is oxygen therapy needed? *Anesth Analg* 1995;**80**:368–72.

5   Sriwatanabul K, Kelvie W, Lasagna L. The quantification of pain: an analysis of words used to describe pain and analgesia in clinical trials. *Clin Pharmacol Ther* 1982;**32**:143–8.

6   Aldrete JA, Kroulik D. A postanesthetic recovery score. *Anesth Analg* 1970;**49**:924–34.

7   Steward DJ. A simplified scoring system for the post-operative recovery room. *Can Anaesth Soc J* 1975;**22**:111–13.

8   Aldrete JA. The post-anesthesia recovery score revisited (letter). *J Clin Anesth* 1995;7:89–91.

9   Watcha MF, White PF. Postoperative nausea and vomiting. Its etiology, treatment, and prevention. *Anesthesiology* 1992;**77**:162–84.

10   Claxton AR, McGuire G, Chung F, Cruise C. Evaluation of morphine versus fentanyl for postoperative analgesia after ambulatory surgical procedures. *Anesth Analg* 1997;**84**:509–14.

11   Tong D, Chung F, Wong D. Predictive factors in global and anesthesia satisfaction in ambulatory surgical patients. *Anesthesiology* 1997;**87**:856–64.

12   Lubarsky DA. Fast track in the post-anesthesia care unit: unlimited possibilities? *J Clin Anesth* 1996;**8**(suppl 3S):70S–72S.

13   Sá Rêgo MM, Watcha MF, White PF. The changing role of Monitored Anesthesia Care in the ambulatory setting. *Anesth Analg* 1997;**85**:1020–36.

14   Song D, Joshi GP, White PF. Fast-track eligibility after ambulatory anesthesia: a comparison of desflurane, sevoflurane, and propofol. *Anesth Analg* 1998;**86**:267–73.

15   White PF. Criteria for fast-tracking outpatients after ambulatory surgery (letter). *J Clin Anesth* 1998;**11**:78–9.

16   Rose DK, Cohen MM. Bypassing the post anaesthetic care unit: cost savings versus patient safety (abstract). *Can J Anaesth* 1996;**43**(suppl):A32-B.

17   Dexter F, Macario A, Manberg PJ, Lubarsky DA. Computer simulation to determine how rapid anesthetic recovery protocols to decrease the time for emergence or increase the Phase I Postanesthesia care unit bypass rate affect staffing of an ambulatory surgery center. *Anesth Analg* 1999;**88**:1053–63.

18   Michaloliakou C, Chung F, Sharma S. Preoperative multimodal analgesia facilitates recovery after ambulatory laparoscopic cholecystectomy. *Anesth Analg* 1996;**82**:44–51.

19   Eriksson H, Tenhunen A, Korttila K. Balanced analgesia improves recovery and outcome after outpatient tubal ligation. *Acta Anaesthesiol Scand* 1996;**40**:151–5.

20   Jin F, Chung F, Norris A, Ganeshram T. Should adult patients drink before discharge from the ambulatory surgery unit? (abstract). *Can J Anaesth* 1998;**45**(suppl):A25-B.

21   Schreiner MS, Nicolson SC, Martin T, Whitney L. Should children drink before discharge from day surgery? *Anesthesiology* 1992;**76**:528–33.

22   Marshall SI, Chung F. Discharge criteria and complications after ambulatory surgery. *Anesth Analg* 1999;**88**:508–17.

23   Marshall S, Chung F. Assessment of 'home readiness': discharge criteria and postdischarge complications. *Curr Opin Anaesthesiol* 1997;**10**:445–50.

24   Korttila K. Recovery from outpatient anaesthesia: factors affecting outcome. *Anaesthesia* 1995;**50**(suppl):22–8.

25   Royal College of Surgeons of England. Commission on the Provision of Surgical Services. *Guidelines for day case surgery*. London: HMSO, 1992.

26   Stott NCH. Day case surgery generates no increased workload for community based staff. True or false? *Br Med J* 1992;**304**:825–6.

27   Elwood JH, Godden S, Barlow J. General practitioners and community staff contacts after day care. *J One-day Surg* 1995;**5**(2):17–18.

28   Roddam PA, Iredale J, Lewis I, Jackson IJB. More expansion of day surgery; a repeat survey of general practitioners' views. *J One-day Surg* 1997;**7**(1):11–16.
29   Jackson IJB, Paton RH, Hawkshaw D. Telephone follow-up the day after day surgery. *J One-day Surg* 1997;**6**(4):5–7.
30   Jackson I. Droperidol–contra-indicated in day surgery? *J One-day Surg* 1999;**8**(4):14–15.
31   Audit Commission. *Measuring quality. The patient's view of day surgery*. London: HMSO, 1991.
32   Ware G. The operational policy and procedures in a hospital hotel. *J One-day Surg* 1993;**3**:9–12.
33   Healy J, Phillips D, Caballero C, Willison J, Souter R, McWhinnie D. The extended day surgery unit (abstract). *J One-day Surg* 1998;**8**(1):22.

9: The paediatric day case

Dori Ann McCulloch

Overview

This chapter aims to revisit most of the topics already discussed in the previous eight chapters, but with the focus clearly on the special needs of children. Many, but not all, of the principles already discussed may be applied to children but most will need to be adapted to meet the different needs of the paediatric day case.

The numerous differences between adults and children will be discussed, not least the additional problems of dealing with both patients and parents. Preassessment will be described and will consider the difficulties in interacting with children of varying ages, the differences in pathology and procedures from those encountered in adults and the additional requirements for emotional and psychological preparation. The particular problems associated with some specific procedures, such as tonsillectomy and chair dental anaesthesia, will be considered.

The provision of premedication, general anaesthesia, perioperative analgesia, and antiemetic therapy for children will be described with appropriate dosage recommendations. Specific problems of maintaining the paediatric airway will be considered. The role of sedation and regional anaesthesia will be discussed. Specific recovery problems and discharge criteria will be covered.

Introduction

Day case surgery for children is not a new concept. Nichol published a series of 8988 children in 1909, which represents one of the first reports of successful day surgery.[1] Children tend to be fit, primarily have minor procedures performed and generally dislike hospitals; therefore they are ideal candidates for day case procedures.

There has been a considerable expansion in day case surgery, both adult and paediatric, over the past few years. This has generally been driven by a desire to cut costs, free hospital beds, and reduce waiting times. Paediatric day surgery conveys the same obvious benefits of cost savings and improved efficiency seen in adults but also offers several advantages for the child.

Children are not adults! There are many differences in the approach to a paediatric patient for day case surgery. In addition, there are significant benefits to be achieved. Minimising the disruption to the child's and family's life is desirable. Children can be very disoriented by unfamiliar surroundings and people and despite improvements in making hospital wards child friendly, they can still be deemed a hostile environment. The emotional and psychological implications of being admitted overnight to the hospital may be severe. Day surgery minimises behavioural problems, disrupted sleep, and enuresis in comparison with inpatient stays.[2] Children tend to mend better at home. Most of the common procedures children undergo tend to be relatively short and non-invasive, associated with minimal blood loss and mild to moderate pain, allowing for convalescence at home without the need for intensive nursing or physiotherapy. Furthermore, children do not harbour preconceived notions regarding recovery lengths or morbidity and so accept the accelerated recovery afforded by day surgery.

Preoperative assessment of the child

Differences from adults

Children are not adults! It may be repeated but it is important to remember. Each of the components of providing anaesthesia to children is different to delivering the same care to an adult. One of the most important differences between adult and paediatric anaesthesia is the involvement of parents, who bring their knowledge, preconceptions, and fears to the child's experience. This can occasionally be helpful. With many parents, however, the feeling of helplessness involved in becoming a patient takes on a life of its own when their children are involved. Therefore, both the patient's and the parents' expectations and anxieties must be dealt with.

Interacting with children
Most children below the age of 12 are unlikely to be able to provide a complete and accurate medical history. Some may not interact with a stranger (e.g. the anaesthetist) at all, despite the use of props and toys. The history will therefore need to be taken from an adult. It is preferable, but not always possible, for this to be the primary caregiver. It is the legal guardian who gives consent for the procedure, not the child and not always the primary caregiver. Therefore the guardian should understand the operation and be able to consent for the operation and anaesthetic.

Because of the range of ages, maturity, and understanding, there are different ways of interacting with children. I believe that a common mistake in dealing with children is to ignore them completely and discuss their condition and the procedure with the parent or guardian. The child is the patient and although they may not be able to communicate effectively, they must not be overlooked. If possible, communication and some sort of rapport should be established with your patient. If nothing further, the child should be greeted in order to let them know that they are important in this process. Asking their age is usually a relatively non-threatening question that most children from the age of three will be able to answer. These things may help them feel more comfortable with you and, possibly, the whole procedure.

Although assessing a child for a day case procedure does not allow you enough time to develop a close or familiar relationship with them, any familiarity cannot hurt. You will be someone else they and their parents recognise. Interacting with the child is important; this is their operation, their lives and, to a certain degree, their choice. Preadmission clinics will help prepare them for the hospital experience.

Psychological preparation

Most of the psychological and emotional preparation for the day case operation will have taken place at home, with varying degrees of success and dependent upon the parents' anxiety level. If children have not been prepared by their parents for the experience of surgery, there is not a great deal that can be done to correct this under the ever-present time constraints on the day of surgery. Many children are unable to express their experiences or feelings in a clear manner, as their frame of reference or vocabulary may be inadequate. This can be a problem both pre- and postoperatively. Understanding that it is a frightening and unfamiliar situation in a hostile environment will provide you with some insight into their fears. This is where the great advantage of preassessment clinics is demonstrable.[3] These prepare the children and the parents for an experience that both will potentially imagine as significantly worse than it will be and can effectively diminish some of their anxieties.

Paediatric preassessment clinics

Nurse-led preassessment clinics for children have become very popular. To minimise disruption for children and parents, these are generally held outside normal school hours, sometimes at weekends. They are therefore often known as "Saturday clubs", although many are actually held on weekday afternoons!

Preadmission clubs allow an opportunity to identify potential anaesthetic or health risks prior to admission. Indeed, much of the preoperative assessment can be performed in a preadmission clinic, which facilitates admitting a large number of patients in a short period of time on the day of surgery and therefore makes the running of the day unit much more efficient. Most importantly, the preassessment club also decreases the parental and child anxiety by introducing the children to the hospital environment, staff, and equipment. It allows ample time for anxiety and fears to be expressed and discussed. The aims of our preadmission programme are listed in Box 9.1.

Box 9.1 The aims of the preadmission programme

- To introduce both child and family to the hospital environment prior to admission.
- To help to make a child's admission to hospital less traumatic and to try to eliminate the fear of the unknown.
- To give parents some knowledge about the child's admission so that they can answer the inevitable questions and "talk it through" with the children.
- To familiarise the children with the equipment, surroundings, and people that they may see while in hospital.
- To reassure parents that we welcome their presence and that we wish to share the care of their children with them and to work together with them to make their child's stay in hospital as pleasant as possible.

Preadmission clinics are generally run by nursing staff but medical staff may also be present and should be contactable to answer specific queries. Typically, children (and their parents) are invited a week or two prior to their admission to be given a tour of the ward, told about the doctors they will interact with and what else they might experience. Both children and parents are given an opportunity to ask questions in a less threatening environment, with fewer time pressures. They are also provided with some anaesthetic equipment (e.g. facemasks and reservoir bags) to play with, so that it becomes more familiar. The information supplied is often supplemented with written material to take home.

There are many advantages to the overall management of the day unit as well. Admission on the day of surgery is hectic, busy, and likely to be slightly chaotic. Children have to be assessed by the nursing staff, anaesthetists, and surgeons. This can be incredibly overwhelming. By having the children attend a preadmission clinic, many of the basic tasks and questions can be dealt with. Weight, blood pressure, and heart rate can be obtained. History questionnaires can be filled out by parents, potentially providing the anaesthetist with important information before the day of surgery. Some difficult problems can be identified and solved before "the big day" arrives. Alternatively, if a problem is detected, the patient may be rescheduled at a more appropriate time, rather than attending the hospital only to be cancelled on the day of surgery.

Selection of surgical procedures

The basic principles underlying the selection of suitable surgical procedures in children are similar to those in adults (Chapter 1). The types of pathology and surgical procedures encountered in children differ from those in adults, however. Congenital abnormalities are relatively common and most defects tend to be corrected early, usually leaving the child clinically unaffected afterwards (e.g. cleft lip or palate). Some conditions may require multiple, follow-up procedures, however. It is less common to encounter acquired pathology in children than in adults, although minor trauma is common. Children may well require anaesthesia for procedures which can easily be performed on conscious adults. A selection of typical paediatric day case procedures is listed in Box 9.2.

Box 9.2 Surgical procedures which are suitable, and typically performed as day cases in children

Ear, nose & throat	Myringotomy tubes, adenoidectomy,* tonsillectomy,* laryngoscopy
Eye surgery	Strabismus (squint) correction, EUA, lacrimal duct probing
Endoscopy	Upper GI endoscopy, colonoscopy, sigmoidoscopy, bronchoscopy
General surgery	Hernia repair (inguinal, epigastric and umbilical), EUA, ingrowing toe nail
Oral surgery	Dental extractions, dental conservation, tongue tie
Orthopaedic	Change of plaster, EUA, peripheral bone and soft tissue surgery, arthroscopy, removal of metalwork
Plastic surgery	Cleft lip, pinnaplasty, skin lesion removal
Urology	Circumcision, division of prepucial adhesions, orchidopexy, hydrocoele repair, minor hypospadias, cystoscopy
Medical	Bone marrow aspiration, lumbar puncture, radiotherapy, imaging, interventional radiology/cardiology, invasive line placement

* Not universally considered suitable for day surgery
EUA, examination under anaesthesia

Day case tonsillectomy
The selection of tonsillectomy (± adenoids) as a day case procedure is still relatively controversial. In many countries, this has long been a day case operation without significant problems. Elsewhere, the major concern is the risk of postoperative bleeding. Bleeding following tonsillectomy follows a well-recognised pattern. Primary bleeding usually occurs within a few hours and should therefore be detectable before a day case patient is discharged. Secondary bleeding, as a result of infection, typically occurs after several days and would therefore not be prevented by an overnight admission.

How late does primary bleeding present? Moralee & Murray used their computerised hospital record system to review a series of 2157 tonsillectomies over a five-year period.[4] During this time there were 42 serious bleeds, of which only 17 were primary. The average time at which patients reentered the operating theatre for reexploration was 2.8 hours (range 0–7, 95% CI of upper limit: 5.2–8.4 h), although it is likely that the *diagnosis* of primary bleeding was made at an earlier time. The authors concluded that day case tonsillectomy should be safe provided that patients were observed for about eight hours.[4] Experience from the United States suggests that discharging children within 5–6 hours of tonsillectomy does not increase the incidence of post discharge complications.[5] Paediatric tonsillectomy is currently included in the British Association of Day Surgery's "trolley" of suitable procedures.[6]

Outpatient dental anaesthesia
Dental anaesthesia is the most common outpatient procedure done in the UK, with approximately 300 000 general anaesthetics administered per year, many of them to children. A substantial number of these procedures are performed in the dental chair, often outside the operating theatre environment, in remote locations not associated with hospitals. The provision of facilities and equipment has often been inadequate and staff may be unfamiliar with the delivery of emergency care. Each year a few potentially preventable deaths occur and there has been a tremendous increase in concern over the safety of chair dental anaesthesia. Several expert bodies have made recommendations for improvements but implementation of these has been variable. Deaths continue to occur, particularly in those under 16 years old, and radical changes have been proposed.[7] It has been suggested that the number of dental general anaesthetics be substantially reduced (the very high numbers appear to be a uniquely British phenomenon), and that the remainder be performed within the hospital setting.[7] A number of hospitals have already established dental facilities following earlier recommendations.[8]

Many of the concepts of providing anaesthesia for major dental procedures in children are similar to those of other day case procedures. Chair dental anaesthesia for more minor procedures (extractions of primary dentition, conservation work) provides many challenges, however. In addition to the location, staff, and equipment, there is often no secured airway and this must be shared with the dentist. Both blood and teeth become at risk of being aspirated by the spontaneously breathing patient. Laryngospasm is a constant possibility. Intravenous access is commonly not obtained. These difficulties would suggest that only the most experienced anaesthetists should provide anaesthesia for chair dental patients. A high degree of suspicion of potential difficulties and good airway management skills are paramount.

Gaseous induction and maintenance of anaesthesia has always been the standard in the dental chair, with halothane being used frequently. Arrhythmias are common during dental extractions and have been suspected as being one of the major causes of death. The incidence of dysrhythmias, especially ventricular, is much lower when sevoflurane is used in place of halothane[9] and this may increase safety. The use of the laryngeal mask may improve airway management and protect against aspiration of blood and debris without impeding surgical access.[10]

Medical assessment

Luckily, most children presenting for day case surgery do not have extremely complex medical conditions or systemic illnesses. Overall, their general health is likely to be good but a complete history and physical examination are necessary in all cases. Although children are generally healthy, special attention should be given to pregnancy and birth difficulties, prematurity, asthma, recent colds, and illnesses. Children who were born prematurely may have a number of chronic illnesses or health problems. These include conditions such as bronchopulmonary dysplasia and other lung pathology or neurological abnormalities, some of which may make them unsuitable for day case procedures.

There are many differences between the airway of a child and that of an adult but the mouth must also not be overlooked. Although it is unusual for children to have caps or crowns, they are very likely to be in some stage of losing "baby" teeth. Teeth begin to become loose from about five, beginning with the incisors, and loose teeth can be a potential difficulty until about 12 years of age. Dislodged teeth are a grave risk to the airways and it is important to establish which teeth are loose, as well as how loose. While discussing the teeth, it is logical to go on to establish the last time the patient ate or drank. This finding is important and may result in postponement of surgery or administration of an oral clear liquid (see later).

Examination of the child
The examination of a paediatric patient may be a challenge. The combination of stranger anxiety, age, cooperation, and your experience with children may prevent you getting a good listen to their chest, much less their heart. If there has been a history of a recent cough, cold or wheezing, the chest should be closely examined. Children with audible pathology are not usually suitable as day cases. As with adults, if the patient can be in better health, it is prudent to postpone the surgical procedure until that time. Most children who are not in excellent health should not be treated as day cases. In most instances, the parents are the best judge of the health of their child. If they feel their child is unwell or not behaving normally (i.e. playing, eating or sleeping), then there will be a better time to anaesthetise them.

Laboratory investigations

As with adults, there are few tests that are of any value for children under-going day case procedures, unless the history specifically dictates them. There may be some benefit from screening children from high-risk popula-tions for sickle cell disease, as symptoms may not yet have presented in young children. As with adults, sickle trait is relatively unimportant as long as good anaesthetic technique is followed. A small number of children who have something in their history to suggest anaemia may require investi-gation. Anaemia may be difficult to detect clinically but most cases that are detected by screening can still undergo day surgery (without correction of blood count) without problems.[11] Even in children who might have physio-logical anaemia of the newborn, haemoglobin concentrations are not routinely indicated.

Specific paediatric problems

In the future, it will not be uncommon to see children with serious but stable medical conditions for day case surgery in locations outside paedi-atric hospitals. In this case it is crucial for the child to be in good general health, despite the co-existing systemic disease or chronic condition, and to fulfil appropriate criteria for day case management. An example may be a child with severe cerebral palsy or seizures who is well, or well controlled, with or without medication. Even children with insulin-dependent diabetes may be possible to treat as day cases. Obviously, the children's hospital with more resources may choose to select children with severe systemic illnesses for day cases, whereas a smaller peripheral hospital will choose to treat them as inpatients or refer them elsewhere. There may not always be a straight-forward answer to these problems and having an accessible bed for admission may allow you to make a decision to proceed, with the option of an overnight stay if necessary.

Congenital diseases

There are a few groups of children in whom it is probably not advisable to carry out day surgery. The first are children with complex congenital heart disease. However, children with uncomplicated lesions, such as atrioseptal defect (ASD), small ventriculoseptal defects (VSD) or asymptomatic surgi-cally corrected defects, may be suitable for day case procedures, provided appropriate antibiotic prophylaxis against bacterial endocarditis is given. Amoxycillin (or clindamycin in hypersensitive individuals) is commonly used but up-to-date advice may be found in current national formularies or from the microbiology department. These children must be otherwise well if they are to be suitable day cases.

A child with an undiagnosed heart murmur is another dilemma. If the child is under one year of age, a cardiological opinion is indicated, as a potentially serious lesion may not yet have become evident. Older children of normal height, weight, and stature, who have an average exercise tolerance and no history of cyanosis or shortness of breath or excessive chest infections, are much less likely to have a serious cardiac anomaly. However, if you are uncomfortable with a newly found murmur, a cardiology evaluation may be advisable before proceeding.

Neonates

Another group of children potentially unsuitable for day case anaesthesia are neonates. Although it may be possible to safely anaesthetise children under two months of age, there are enough risk factors to suggest that safety may require an overnight stay. Typically, infants under the age of 50 weeks postconceptual age are not considered suitable for day case procedures, due to an increased risk of postoperative apnoea.[12,13] The former preterm infant is also more likely to experience inadequate temperature control and may have continuing respiratory problems in addition to their immature respiratory centres. Bronchopulmonary dysplasia, previous apnoea, and concurrent physiological anaemia may make them even poorer candidates for day case surgery.

Anaesthetists or centres that do not routinely work with infants or neonates may choose to have a lower age limit of six months (or even a year) for day case procedures, except possibly for examinations under anaesthesia. Erring on the side of caution is a prudent practice for these patients. If the centre and clinicians are familiar with neonates, they may choose to attempt more procedures. Luckily, there are not many under one-year-olds attending for straightforward day case procedures.

Common preoperative problems

Upper respiratory tract infection

Despite thorough and careful preadmission assessment, new developments can occur by the day of admission. The most common problem is the child with a recent, or current, upper respiratory illness.

There is no easy or pat answer. Because children have very reactive airways, it is advantageous to avoid acute illnesses that may compound the potential for laryngospasm or bronchospasm. Increased airway reactivity may persist for up to six weeks following acute upper respiratory tract infections (URTIs).[14] Despite this, in practice serious perioperative complications are relatively uncommon and generally mild in patients with URTIs.[14]

In deciding on the management of the child with a URTI, the question that should be asked is, "Can this child be in a significantly better state of health?". If your answer is "yes", then the patient should be sent home to achieve that state. Children who are clinically unwell or toxic should definitely be postponed, as should children with an elevated temperature. A productive or persistent, non-clearing cough would also suggest a delay. Any wheezing should definitely be corrected before anaesthetising a child. In addition, with decreasing age of the child I would have less inclination to accept potential airway complications. I would think carefully about any child under two years of age with a URTI and would almost certainly defer a child under the age of one year. Because the cellular changes after an upper respiratory illness take 6 to 8 weeks to return to normal,[14] if surgery is to be postponed, it should be for this length of time. Although this is a long time, an elective procedure is just that, *elective*, and there is no need to increase the risk of surgery or anaesthesia unnecessarily in otherwise healthy children.

The child with a runny nose

Not all upper respiratory symptoms suggest URTI and there are procedures performed in the day case setting that may be somewhat curative. These include grommet insertion, adenoidectomy, and tonsillectomy. A persistent cough from postnasal discharge or nasal drainage may accompany the pathology with which these children present for surgery. In this case, a greater tolerance is required for a condition that may improve after surgery. If the parents think that their child is as healthy as possible, that the nose is always dripping, and the child does not appear toxic, then I will often proceed. Because I believe in a safe margin of cynicism, I also ask if the child has been playing, sleeping, and eating normally. If they have, then I usually agree to anaesthetise the child.

After anaesthetising hundreds of children in varying states of illnesses and health, I recognise that many children have a chronic nasal drainage during much of the year without symptoms that parents will admit. Other children have a continually running nose with a cough. There are certain seasons of the year where the number of children with subclinical nasal drainage from either allergies or colds approaches 100%. All these children I would anaesthetise carefully. They are more likely to have a reactive airway, most problematically causing laryngospasm or bronchospasm. The majority of adverse events occurring are not life threatening, however, and can be dealt with by a competent anaesthetist familiar with children. Avoiding instrumentation of the larynx (by the use of facemask or laryngeal mask) also appears to reduce intraoperative problems.[14,15]

Ultimately, the definition of URTI is as diverse as the presentation of the illness and the science backing the study of URTI and anaesthesia is somewhat lacking. Therefore much of the decision is based upon clinical judgement and skill in dealing with paediatric patients. There must be clear communication with the surgeon and parents detailing the potential increased risk of airway-related complications in children who have upper respiratory symptoms.

Paediatric day care facilities

Although children and adults can be managed in the same surgical day unit, special considerations must be given to the children's comfort. There are significant differences in the support and care of children, therefore paediatric specialists need to create a child-friendly environment.

How is the management of children different from that of adults? Children may not have the verbal skills or understanding that an adult has and may imagine a scenario far worse than that which they ultimately experience. There has been much speculation on the reasons why young children are particularly vulnerable to the hospital experience. The limitations imposed on the child by their cognitive development level and lack of worldly experience contribute to making the hospital a totally unfamiliar and unpredictable environment.

Children should be given a place that has distractions and an environment which are suitable for the ages operated upon. Assessment of children's behaviour, both before and after surgery, is best done by staff able to understand their needs and appropriately trained to do so. Children often do not ask for pain relief, so the staff must be able to assess subtle clues and be trained to use age-appropriate paediatric pain-scoring systems. Both staff and patients enjoy the cheery environments created especially for kids. Having the ability to amuse themselves with specially provided games, toys, televisions, and videos may distract children and lessen their preoperative anxiety.

It could be argued that a day case unit that only sees an occasional child should not do paediatric work at all. The many differences between children and adults mean that complications and treatments are not the same and the lack of paediatric experience may put the child at a greater risk. Places that see more than the occasional child should be able to provide at least one paediatric-trained member of staff.

It is also important to remember that the equipment utilised for children is different. An adequate supply of all equipment, both for routine care and for the treatment of emergencies, must be available (Box 9.3). This in itself can make it less cost-effective to provide day case surgery for the occasional child. All staff working in paediatric day care must be familiar with paediatric resuscitation. Specific guidelines change from time to time and the reader is referred to the current national recommendations of their country. Typical doses of some of the more common emergency paediatric drugs are listed in Table 9.1.

Preparation for surgery

Fasting guidelines

Fasting has been given a lot of consideration over the last decade. Although there are some differences in opinion, most clinicians would agree that it is

Box 9.3 Some of the equipment required for paediatric day case anaesthesia. The exact requirements will depend on the age range of children and the complexity of surgical procedures selected

Airway management:	Selection of laryngeal masks Facemasks of different shapes and sizes, preferably scented Range of oral and nasal airways Range of cuffed and non-cuffed tracheal tubes and connectors Variety of laryngoscope blades, including straight Small diameter tubing and 1 litre bag to modify circle system (consider T-piece for very small children) Paediatric suction catheters
Fluid management:	20, 22 and 24 G intravenous cannulae Infusion tubing with minimal deadspace Paediatric fluid administration sets (Consider need for volumetric pumps)
Temperature:	Warming blanket or forced air blower Paediatric fluid warmers (Consider heated humidification of inspired gas) Paediatric temperature probes
Monitoring:	Paediatric pulse oximeter probes Range of blood pressure cuffs Paediatric electrocardiograph electrodes Appropriate sampling rate on gas/volatile agent monitor
Recovery and emergency:	Paediatric oxygen masks Defibrillator with paediatric paddles Appropriate sizes of "difficult airway" equipment Paediatric self-inflating bag Range of resuscitation drugs in appropriate dose

Table 9.1 Selection of drugs and appropriate doses for use in paediatric resuscitation and other emergencies. Defibrillation energies are also given. Practitioners should be familiar with current paediatric resuscitation guidelines

Drug	Dose	Comments
Epinephrine (adrenaline)	Initial 10 µg/kg Subsequent 100 µg/kg	0.1 ml/kg of 1 in 10 000 0.1 ml/kg of 1 in 1000 (use 10 x dose via tracheal tube if no intravenous access)
Atropine	20 µg/kg	Dilute to 100 µg/ml and give 0.2 ml/kg
Diazepam	200–300 µg/kg	Respiratory depression likely
Naloxone	10 µg/kg	Increase dose if no response
Fluid bolus	20 ml/kg crystalloid or colloid	Assess response, repeat if necessary
Defibrillation	First 2 shocks 2 J/kg Subsequent shocks 4 J/kg	Anterior-posterior paddle configuration

safe to administer clear fluids until two hours before anaesthesia and solids until six hours before an anaesthetic.[16, 17] The complications for children are how to classify breast milk and formula. Most breastfed infants are fed every 3-4 hours and the stomach is likely to be empty before each feed. The consensus view is that breast milk is safe up to four hours before induction of anaesthesia but that formula and other non-human milk should be considered as solids and withheld for six hours.[18]

Ideally, children should no longer be fasted from midnight until their morning position on an operating list. Children probably have a lower incidence of hypotension or hypoglycaemia perioperatively if they receive appropriate preoperative fluids but this has not been adequately studied. Although it is not fair to have children woken up for a drink in the middle of the night, parents could be asked to provide a drink of a sugar-containing solution before coming into the hospital on the day of surgery. Since the majority of patients will have to leave the house approximately two hours before the start of the operating list to make their way to the hospital for any further admission proceedings, this should not be a problem. The instructions must be clear, so that toast does not join the liquid! Children who are not first on the operating list could also be offered clear liquid on arrival if they are likely to be two hours away from their procedure.

Premedication

To premedicate or not to premedicate, that is the question. My answer changes every so often depending upon the prevailing winds! There are a few difficulties with premedication in the day case setting. The first is the organisation of timing, the second is the duration of action, the third is variability of effect (occasionally adverse), and the last, for my favourite premedication, is the taste.

Oral midazolam

If a sedative premedication is required, oral midazolam is probably the best choice and has achieved popularity for a number of reasons. Orally administered midazolam (0.5 mg/kg) takes 15–20 minutes to work, does not usually have a prolonged (postoperative) sedative effect and is a very effective amnestic. The parenteral preparation of midazolam is used and, unfortunately, its taste is disgusting. Subsequently, it is difficult to convince a small child that the postoperative painkillers will not taste the same as the premedication. The taste can be masked somewhat by giving midazolam in a sugar (or concentrated juice) solution or placing it in combination with a paracetamol (acetaminophen) or non-steroidal antiinflammatory syrup. This may have the added benefit of providing prophylactic analgesia (see later). In the USA, a new commercial oral formulation of midazolam has become available, although it is more expensive than the parenteral preparation.

219

Other measures to reduce anxiety

Even with its rapid onset, oral midazolam has to be administered at the appropriate time. Too early and the effect can wear off before induction of anaesthesia; too late and it may not be effective. Other sedative premedications, such as chloral hydrate, temazepam, and triclofos, have a slower onset of action and provide even bigger timing challenges. Some have a longer lasting effect as well, making them undesirable for day cases. A selection of paediatric sedative premedicants, with suggested doses, is listed in Table 9.2.

Table 9.2 Routine sedative premedication is not recommended for paediatric day cases. If premedication is considered desirable for an individual case, the following may be used

Drug	Dose	Comments
Midazolam	0.25–0.5 mg/kg	Maximum 15–20 mg. Preferred choice, bitter taste
Chloral hydrate	30–50 mg/kg	Maximum 1 g
Triclofos	25–30 mg/kg	0–12 months
	250–500 mg	1–5 years
	0.5–1.0 g	6–12 years

Some investigators have shown that the preoperative interview is as effective as a premedicant in adults.[19] I believe that this should be the case to a certain degree in children as well. If you can familiarise yourself with the patient, it may help to alleviate their anxieties. There are many potential opportunities for your dormant creative side in providing distractions for the patient during induction. You may even be able to play a counting game or use some other tricks to distract or relax the child.

Other forms of premedication

Premedication includes all medication given in the preoperative period, not just those used to produce sedation or relief of anxiety. Any important regular medication which the child is chronically receiving (e.g. bronchodilators) should be taken as normal. In addition, medication may be given to reduce the pain of intravenous cannulation, for postoperative pain relief and, occasionally, for prevention of postoperative nausea and vomiting (PONV).

Topical analgesia

All children who wish to have an intravenous induction of anaesthesia should receive one of the topical local anaesthetic mixtures well before cannula insertion. Both topical amethocaine (Ametop®) and EMLA are suitable. These preparations are probably equally effective if applied for an adequate amount of time. Amethocaine has a faster onset of action, however, and resulted in a higher percentage of pain-free needle insertions compared to EMLA when these preparations were applied to children for 40 minutes.[20] If the patient is first on the operating list, the "magic cream" should be placed as soon as they arrive on the ward, as prearranged. An alternative is to send home local anaesthetic cream from the preadmission clinic for the parents to administer before arriving. Whoever applies the topical anaesthetic must be able to recognise suitable veins for potential cannulation, rather than just applying the cream to "the usual place". Application to two different sites may be advisable if first-time cannulation cannot be guaranteed.

Prophylactic analgesia

The use of analgesics as a "premedicant" in day surgery has widened over the last few years and has an important role to play. Most paediatric day case procedures should not be exceptionally painful, by definition, and the pain should generally be controlled with oral medications. Because drugs like paracetamol and NSAIDs take a reasonable amount of time to become effective, administering them upon recovery, or even intraoperatively (e.g. by suppository), will be too late to prevent pain upon awakening. Giving these drugs prophylactically, by mouth, in the preoperative period should ensure an adequate effect by the end of surgery. This analgesic premedication may often be the only pain relief needed if local anaesthesia is also administered intraoperatively (see later).

Parental presence at induction of anaesthesia

Since most hospitals and anaesthetists have agreed to let parents accompany the children to the anaesthetic room (or to where the induction takes place), the need for (sedative) premedication has diminished. Studies have suggested that the parent's presence is only helpful in a small proportion of cases, however. Anxiety in children was only reduced by parental presence at induction if the child was already calm, if the parent demonstrated low anxiety levels and if the child was more than four years old.[21] In children under four, parental presence may actually increase anxiety.[21] In a follow-up study, both parental presence and midazolam premedication improved the cooperation of children during induction, although premedication was superior and was the only intervention which appeared to reduce the child's anxiety.[21] Nevertheless, parents do provide some familiarity and security to the child. It is important to remember why the parent is there and their presence should not be a right. They are there for the child, to give support, comfort and a degree of familiarity to the unfamiliar environment. Most parents believe that their presence helps the child but this opinion is not shared by many anaesthetists!.[21, 22]

In order to receive the maximum benefit from parents at induction, they need a bit of instruction, as they are often unaware of their purpose. In addition, having an anaesthetic is not like going to sleep. Parents should be informed that purposeful or excitatory movement, eyes rolling to the back of the head and some airway noises are normal for children undergoing induction of anaesthesia. The more information you can provide a parent with, the better they will behave in the induction room. This should decrease their emotional trauma as well. I always ask the parents to hold the child's hand as this provides the benefit of touch to the child and gives the parent something concrete to do and focus on. Most parents find the experience during induction upsetting, although this is diminished on subsequent occasions.[22]

Management of anaesthesia

Inhalational or intravenous induction?

As previously suggested, I believe children should have a choice about how they "go to sleep". There are advantages and disadvantages to both intravenous and inhalational induction (see Table 9.3). With the advent of sevoflurane, which is sweet smelling and not irritating to the airway, there is no reason not to give children a choice and a small amount of control by providing that choice. Most children have a definite preference. Both induction techniques should be familiar to the accomplished practitioner.

Table 9.3 Advantages and disadvantages of inhalational and intravenous induction of anaesthesia

Advantages	Disadvantages
Intravenous induction	
• No facemask required	• Painful
• Intravenous access secured before induction of anaesthesia	• Relatively expensive unless drug ampoules are shared between patients
Inhaled induction	
• Provides supplemental oxygenation	• No intravenous access during induction
• Painless	• Potential for environmental pollution
• Spontaneous ventilation maintained	• Dislike of mask on face

Inhalation induction
Halothane was previously the drug of choice for inhalation induction in children. Sevoflurane, which is less soluble and more pleasant to breathe, has now largely displaced halothane. Inhalation induction with sevoflurane is faster[23] and more pleasant[24] compared to halothane. The lack of airway irritation with sevoflurane allows it to be initiated at 8% without provoking coughing or breath holding. This more rapid induction technique permits faster loss of consciousness, typically about one minute,[24] and also largely eliminates the transient excitement which is often observed with a step-wise

induction technique.[25] Induction with 8% sevoflurane facilitates tracheal intubation within approximately 150 seconds.[26]

Inhalation induction with sevoflurane appears to be very well tolerated, with few complications. Bradycardia has been reported in young children (≤2 years),[27] but does not seem to occur in older children. Respiratory complications are rare and generally mild, even in children with respiratory tract infections.[28] There is no place for induction with enflurane, isoflurane or desflurane, which are highly irritant and offer no advantage over sevoflurane.

Intravenous induction
Either through dislike of masks and smells or for other reasons, some children prefer an intravenous induction. The prior application of topical anaesthesia and a good technique should make this relatively painless. While any intravenous induction agent could potentially be used, propofol is the drug of choice for similar reasons to those in adults (Chapter 4).

Compared to adults, the volume of propofol's central compartment (on a per kilogram basis) is larger and clearance is also higher.[29] Consequently, the induction dose required in children is considerably greater than it is in adults, with doses of at least 2.5–3 mg/kg being needed.

Propofol is generally well tolerated in children. Induction produces a decrease in both heart rate and blood pressure, although rarely to a clinically significant degree. The most common problem is pain on injection of propofol. This may be relieved to some degree by the addition of lidocaine (lignocaine), although quite a large dose, sometimes as much as 40 mg, may be required.[30] Despite lidocaine, some children still find propofol painful.

Maintenance of anaesthesia

Maintenance of anaesthesia is still primarily inhalation based in children. Less soluble anaesthetics, such as desflurane and sevoflurane, offer the advantage of more rapid emergence and, in some cases, earlier discharge times. Because desflurane is so unsuitable for inhalation induction in children, it does not appear to have become popular for maintenance either. Sevoflurane is a more logical choice, being a natural follow-on from the induction phase.

Unfortunately, sevoflurane has been associated with several reports of excitement occurring during the emergence phase. This is not just a property of sevoflurane and may be a feature of all rapidly eliminated anaesthetics. Indeed, emergence excitement is even more common after desflurane anaesthesia.[31] The exact cause of this excitement is not known. There is no doubt that rapid recovery from anaesthesia will unmask pain if it is present and inadequate early analgesia probably explains at least some cases of "excitement".[32] This is not the whole story, however, and excitement is still observed in apparently pain-free children. Although post-operative agitation is unpleasant to observe and may be time consuming for recovery staff, it is generally self-limiting and does not result in any obvious after-effects in the happy children usually observed 2–3 hours after the end of anaesthesia.

Anaesthesia may also be maintained by an infusion of propofol, although this technique is less common in children than in adults. Infusions of propofol have been associated with adverse outcomes in very young children receiving it as a sedative in the intensive care unit.[33] There appears to be much less risk when propofol is used during anaesthesia, although in the UK it is not licensed as a maintenance agent in children less than three years old (although licensed for induction in infants over one month).

Because of a larger central compartment volume and greater clearance, children will require maintenance infusion rates 25–50% higher than those in adults. Target-controlled infusion (TCI) systems currently use adult pharmacokinetic values. Applying these to children will produce plasma concentrations somewhat lower than those intended, with a discrepancy which varies over time.[34] For this reason, the commercial TCI system should not be used in children and will not permit the entry of an age less than 16 years. Paediatric pharmacokinetic models may become commercially available in the future.

As in adults, propofol anaesthesia facilitates rapid emergence and is associated with a reduction in PONV.[35, 36] Propofol infusions can be especially useful in children potentially susceptible to malignant hyperpyrexia.

Management of the airway

The laryngeal mask airway
With the introduction of the laryngeal mask airway (LMA), there is hardly any need for an alternative airway for day case surgery. Many of the advantages of the LMA are self-evident but there are particular benefits in day surgery. The LMA avoids instrumenting the airway, which may be especially desirable in children with upper respiratory infections[15] or asthma. The LMA requires a lighter plane of anaesthesia for airway placement[37] and maintenance[38] compared to a tracheal tube. It also allows for elimination of neuromuscular blocking drugs and reversal agents, facilitating spontaneous breathing. Spontaneous ventilation anaesthesia offers greater flexibility; there is no need to try to predict when the operation will end, as with repeated doses of neuromuscular blocking agents. Spontaneous ventilation is also safer in the event of a breathing circuit disconnection, while the breathing rate and pattern give some guide to the anaesthetic depth.

Although not a perfect airway, the LMA ought to be suitable for most paediatric day case procedures, where patients are healthy and appropriately fasted. The LMA offers excellent protection of the airway from contamination by blood and debris coming from above and may therefore have particular advantages in oral and pharyngeal operations. For example, during adenotonsillectomy, the LMA provided superior protection of the trachea from blood and consequently reduced postoperative stridor and coughing, compared to a tracheal tube.[39] Not intubating the trachea in children undergoing adenoidectomy, who often have low-grade, chronic respiratory tract infections, is probably advantageous.[15] The LMA is also useful in dental surgery and avoids the epistaxis associated with nasal intubation.[40]

Although the LMA is used routinely in paediatric patients, it must be remembered that it is not always as effective an airway in children as in adults. Problems with the LMA, including difficulty in placement, partial obstruction, and activation of airway reflexes, occur with an overall incidence of approximately 20% but are more common with small-sized LMAs and with less experienced anaesthetists.[41] Despite this high frequency of airway-related problems, most difficulties are relatively easy to overcome and do not result in significant morbidity, making the LMA a safe and effective airway.[41]

There is mixed evidence as to whether it is more advantageous to remove the laryngeal mask when the paediatric patient is awake[42] or deeply anaesthetised.[43] Clinically, waiting for the return of protective airway reflexes with the LMA in place demonstrates no significant ill effects and has the advantage of not having to manually support the airway or disturb the awakening child.

Tracheal intubation and neuromuscular block
Where intubation of the trachea is required for surgical access or other indications, this can be facilitated by the use of a short-acting neuromuscular blocking agent. Succinylcholine (suxamethonium) was previously popular but its use is commonly associated with arrhythmias.[44] More serious cardiac complications may also occur,[45] and it has been recommended that succinylcholine should not be used routinely in children.[46] None of the non-depolarising neuromuscular blocking drugs are ideal alternatives; rocuronium is rapid acting but of moderate duration, whereas mivacurium has short (and highly variable) duration but slow onset and also releases histamine. The best choice will depend upon the exact circumstances of each individual case.

Another alternative is to intubate the trachea under deep anaesthesia, but without neuromuscular block. One approach is to use propofol (3–4 mg/kg) and alfentanil (15 µg/kg),[47] while another is to use 8% sevoflurane.[26] In direct comparisons performed in children, both techniques produced tracheal intubating conditions which were subtly inferior to those achieved with succinylcholine (1.5–2 mg/kg), but which were nevertheless clinically acceptable. Achieving tracheal intubation without neuromuscular block has the added advantages that spontaneous ventilation will recommence sooner (especially with an inhalational technique) and the risk of inadequate reversal is eliminated. The possibility of abnormal pseudocholinesterases (which alter the metabolism of succinylcholine and mivacurium) also becomes irrelevant.

Fluids

The administration of intravenous fluids during day case surgery is still uncommon in the United Kingdom. The benefits of such therapy are still controversial, although some evidence suggests an improved outcome with fluid administration. In adults, 20 ml/kg of an electrolyte solution reduced postoperative drowsiness, dizziness, and nausea for up to a day after surgery.[48] There may be an advantage to administering a balanced salt solution to young children fasted for a prolonged time, children undergoing procedures associated with a high incidence of PONV or procedures with increased incidence of perioperative haemorrhage. A reduced preoperative fluid fast should also help.

Monitoring

Appropriate monitoring is just as important in paediatric day cases as it is in all other forms of anaesthesia. Full monitoring to the appropriate national standards must always be used. The case for temperature monitoring should be considered carefully. Malignant hyperpyrexia is rare and the incidence of dramatic cases is likely to decrease as succinylcholine and halothane are used less. Hypothermia is more likely, however, as small children have a greater surface area than adults and are therefore more likely to lose heat, even during short procedures.

Role of regional anaesthesia and/or sedation in children

There are a number of small procedures which, in adults, might be performed under sedation, with local infiltration or with no anaesthesia at all. These include radiological procedures (e.g. MRI, CT), radiotherapy, lumbar puncture, endoscopies, and small lesion removal. Unfortunately, in children these are unlikely to be tolerated without at least a reasonable degree of sedation. There is much confusion involved in clarifying which procedures are suitable for sedation in children and which clinicians are competent to administer it. Because of the difficulties in sedating a child sufficiently, a strong argument has been made for the involvement of an anaesthetist whenever and wherever sedation is needed. Because small children are frightened, cannot understand the need to keep still or are simply unable to do so, the sedation required is significant and rapidly approaches an anaesthetic. In addition, many sedatives have long-lasting effects on patients, whereas giving a child a short anaesthetic with short-acting drugs (such as sevoflurane or propofol) will often allow them to be up and running in a very quick time. The importance of having a professional trained and competent in airway management and resuscitation cannot be overestimated in decreasing morbidity and mortality and has been pointed out on numerous occasions.

Some older children may be more cooperative and may undergo surgery under regional anaesthesia or sedation in much the same way as adults (see Chapter 6).

Anaesthesia outside the operating room

Although most day surgery is performed in an appointed operating theatre, there are a significant number of anaesthetics given in "hostile" environments. This is especially the case in paediatric practice, where anaesthesia is often required for imaging, diagnostic, and radiotherapy procedures. Many of these may be considered day case procedures. Providing a safe anaesthetic outside the operating theatre environment can be a challenge. There are many important considerations, including hazards of the location, the need for special equipment, special requirements (e.g. for MRI scanning) and the availability of ancillary or support staff. Adequate preparation and familiarity with the procedure, location, and equipment are fundamental to safety and success. The specific problems of chair dental anaesthesia were discussed earlier. Further information on other remote locations can be retrieved from textbooks addressing this topic.[49]

Perioperative analgesia

One of the most important aspects of day case anaesthesia is the provision of adequate analgesia. This is especially true in paediatric practice, as a child in pain will rapidly lose confidence in all their carers. The combination of paracetamol, NSAID, and local anaesthetics should provide effective relief of pain for the majority of patients undergoing day case procedures. In particular, opioids should be avoided whenever possible, in order to decrease sedation and side effects, most importantly PONV, which can delay discharge unnecessarily or require admission. If a procedure is going to be exceptionally painful, it is almost certainly not appropriate as a day case. If necessary, a shorter acting opioid such as fentanyl ought to be the first choice. This should not prolong recovery significantly if no side effects are experienced.

In order to ensure that adequate analgesia is provided from the moment the child awakens, at least one analgesic (i.e. NSAID or paracetamol) should be administered *before* the operation begins, with the other being used as a postoperative supplement. It has been recommended to use a relatively high loading dose of paracetamol (e.g. 20 mg/kg orally; 30–45 mg/kg rectally) before following with more standard dosing.[50] Typical paediatric doses of suitable analgesics are shown in Table 9.4.

Table 9.4 *Suitable analgesic medications to use in paediatric day case patients. For procedures expected to produce postoperative pain, at least one analgesic should be administered before induction of anaesthesia*

Drug	Dose	Duration	Comments
Ibuprofen	5–8 mg/kg	4–6 hours	Maximum 40 mg/kg per day
Paracetamol			Maximum 90 mg/kg per day
oral	15 mg/kg	4–6 hours	20 mg/kg loading dose
rectal	20 mg/kg	6–8 hours	30–45 mg/kg loading dose
Codeine	0.5 mg/kg	6 hours	More likely to cause nausea
Bupivacaine infiltration	2 mg/kg	6–8 hours	Volume depends on wound size, use 0.5% if dose limit permits

Local and regional anaesthesia

Although children may not tolerate surgery under local or regional anaesthesia alone, local anaesthetics are incredibly useful for postoperative analgesia and can be used in a number of ways. These include regional nerve block, local infiltration, and topical application.

Regional anaesthesia can be a useful adjunct to general anaesthetic techniques in paediatric day case surgery. A variety of regional nerve blocks can be performed by the anaesthetist for procedures on the arms, legs, abdomen, and genitalia. Further details may be found in major textbooks or a useful recent review.[51] Some of the most common nerve blocks include inguinal nerve block for hernias and orchidopexy, caudal block for hernias or circumcision and dorsal penile nerve block for circumcision. These techniques are summarised in Table 9.5.

When planning to provide a regional technique for a child, it is important to let them know that their arm or legs will feel numb, or different, for a

Table 9.5 *The three most common regional anaesthetic blocks for providing postoperative analgesia in children. Note that in many cases, less invasive techniques may provide comparable analgesia, (see text for details).*

Block	Indication(s)	Anaesthetic	Volume	Comments
Caudal	Circumcision Hernia Feet, legs and toes	Bupivacaine 0.25%	0.8 ml/kg	Especially useful for bilateral procedures
Dorsal nerve of penis	Circumcision	Bupivacaine 0.5%	1 ml + 0.1 ml/kg	Bilateral injection preferable to midline
Ilioinguinal/ iliohypogastric	Inguinal hernia, orchidopexy	Bupivacaine 0.25%	0.25 ml/kg	Best performed with short-bevelled needle

while after surgery but that this is normal and will wear off. Otherwise, you may cause unnecessary distress and concern to a child who didn't entirely understand the surgical process in the first place.

There are special considerations to regional anaesthesia in the day case setting. A significant advantage of regional techniques for major operative procedures is the length of pain relief they can provide. But this extended action can also hamper recovery times, especially for central blocks such as spinals, epidurals, and caudals. The postoperative course may be substantially delayed by prolonged motor block, as well as by sympathetic block, although the latter is less of a problem than it is in adults. Nevertheless, it is possible to use regional techniques combined with general anaesthesia to provide postoperative pain relief without greatly prolonging hospital stay. Some of the techniques employed to minimise morbidity and increase duration of block utilise lower concentrations of local anaesthetic combined with small doses of opioids (fentanyl 1–2 μg/kg), clonidine (1–2 μg/kg) or ketamine (0.5 mg/kg).[52]

Another advantage of regional anaesthetic techniques is the ability to provide effective widespread analgesia with a relatively small dose of local anaesthetic. This may be especially advantageous for bilateral procedures. For example, although simple wound infiltration may be effective for a procedure such as orchidopexy (which may involve bilateral groin and scrotal incisions), it may be difficult to inject a sufficient volume of local anaesthetic into all the wounds, while staying within a total dose of 2 mg/kg of bupivacaine in a small child. Where there is only a single incision, however, wound infiltration may be as effective as a regional block and is simpler and generally safer. An example would be inguinal hernia repair, where wound infiltration has been shown to be as effective as ilioinguinal and iliohypogastric nerve block.[53]

Topical application of local anaesthetics may also be useful after some procedures. Examples include cosmetic procedures and squint repair. Following circumcision, topical application of lidocaine jelly provides equally effective analgesia compared to a dorsal nerve block.[54] Furthermore, topical lidocaine is completely non-invasive and can be reapplied later for prolonged pain relief, a distinct advantage over nerve blocks. Similarly, topical amethocaine eye drops have been shown to provide excellent analgesia after strabismus surgery.[55] Logical advice would be to use the most simple form of local anaesthetic application whenever possible, resorting to invasive and more complex peripheral and central nerve blocks only where they can be shown to provide a distinct advantage.

Recovery

Postoperative care and discharge requirements have progressed over the last few years. In day case surgery, the objectives will be to return the child to their preanaesthetic state as quickly as possible, while attending to discomfort and distress caused by the surgery. Waking up in a child-friendly environment with paediatric support staff can ease some of the anxiety of the postoperative period. Parents can be introduced back to their children as soon as it is possible. Some units allow parents to sit with their children in the recovery room. This may provide both the parents and the children with some anxiety relief, especially if the parents have been well prepared for what to expect.

Pain management

Pain relief will be an important consideration and procedures which are known to be painful should have analgesia administered early, both in and out of the operating theatre, to prevent excessive discomfort. There should not be a need for strong opioids postoperatively for most day case procedures, so providing adequate pain relief should not delay discharge. With the combination of preoperative NSAIDs, local anaesthetic administered intraoperatively and then oral paracetamol and NSAIDs postoperatively, most pain should be adequately controlled. Because children don't express their pain in the same way that adults do, various pain assessments have been developed for children. All have various advantages and disadvantages but whichever system is utilised, pain control should be assessed repeatedly in response to analgesic interventions. It is important to educate both nursing staff and parents about the importance of giving regular analgesia. Providing analgesia on a regular, prophylactic basis, rather than waiting for a child to become excessively uncomfortable, will provide better outcomes.[50]

Postoperative nausea and vomiting

Postoperative nausea and vomiting (PONV) still remains the most significant morbidity experienced by patients after an anaesthetic and is the most common cause of unanticipated admission in children.[56] Unfortunately, many of the common paediatric day case procedures (e.g. strabismus surgery, adenotonsillectomy, prominent ear correction) are associated with high incidences of PONV.

Being able to accurately identify the child at risk, as well as the procedure, will help in the management of PONV. Children at risk include those with a history of motion sickness or PONV. The principles of preventing and treating PONV in children are similar to those in adults (Chapter 7). Basic strategies include avoiding excessive preoperative fasting, intraoperative administration of fluids and discouraging too early postoperative oral intake and mobilisation.

As mentioned previously, the anaesthetic technique can be modified to exclude opioids and possibly neostigmine and nitrous oxide. TIVA with propofol has shown a decreased incidence of PONV in high-risk, strabismus surgery.[57] Most commonly used antiemetics (e.g. metoclopramide, cyclizine, droperidol) have either low efficacy or unpleasant side effects and therefore have no routine place in day case surgery. For the child at risk for PONV, either ondansetron (0.1 mg/kg) or low-dose droperidol (20 μg/kg) may be of use.[58]

Discharge criteria

Anaesthetic, surgical, social, and clinical signs are involved in deciding an appropriate discharge time for children after day case surgery. In the past, the ability to tolerate fluids was an important determination of fitness for discharge. Passing urine has also previously been used as an essential milestone. Critical review of these formal discharge criteria has suggested that some of them may be unnecessary, however. Forcing oral fluids on unwilling children does not appear to improve the outcome following discharge and may actually increase the risk of PONV.[59] Similarly, waiting for the patient to pass urine may simply delay discharge, especially if the child has had nothing to drink. Urinary retention is rare, even when patients are discharged without voiding.[60] Although urinary retention may be more likely after a regional anaesthetic block (e.g. caudals), it is still rare in children.[61] A study comparing caudal and inguinal blocks showed no difference between the groups in the occurrence of urinary retention.[62]

Potentially more important is the achievement of adequate pain relief and the ability to adequately control the pain at home. Although oral analgesics will be used most frequently, there are a few topical preparations that may be helpful (e.g. lidocaine jelly for circumcision pain). Most importantly, parents should be educated that analgesia is essential and should be provided before pain is significant. Prescribing analgesics on a scheduled basis for the first 48 hours should prevent much of the discomfort reported at home immediately postoperatively.

Patients in general should not be discharged home actively vomiting. However, if the child has been adequately hydrated perioperatively, with the fluid deficit replaced, it may be possible to send them home, provided there is appropriate support and understanding and the ability to return to the hospital if the child's condition deteriorates or the vomiting does not resolve overnight.

Instructions to the parents must be clear and provided in both verbal and written formats. Parents must know about postoperative pain relief, diet, and resumption of normal activities. Telephone numbers should be included where parents can seek advice. Calling the families the day after surgery allows further instructions to be given if necessary, provides reassurance to the families and allows complications to be detected. This follow-up will aid in auditing the adequacy of postoperative pain management, frequency of PONV, and surgical morbidity.

Summary

Day case surgery for children is advantageous to the patients, their families, and their health providers in many ways. The need for optimum selection, preparation, and management of anaesthesia is of the utmost importance, as is the requirement for providing anaesthesia and analgesia which will minimise common morbidity. Successful provision of day case services is dependent on these factors. All those involved in paediatric day surgery must be fully aware of the specific needs, problems, pathologies, procedures, techniques, and dose requirements associated with children of varying ages.

Improved anaesthetic techniques, newer short-acting anaesthetic agents and, occasionally, improved surgical techniques all help to return children to their presurgical state as rapidly as possible. This and providing a service causing little postoperative morbidity (i.e. nausea and vomiting or inadequate pain control), few unexpected inpatient admissions and patient and family satisfaction are the goals which all day case providers must try to achieve.

The most rewarding aspect of paediatric day case surgery is visiting the child in the postoperative period and finding them happily playing in the play room.

1   Nicoll JH. The surgery of infancy. *Br Med J* 1909;2:753–4.
2   Scaife JM, Johnstone JM. Psychological aspects of daycare surgery for children. In: Healy TE, ed. *Anaesthesia for day case surgery*. London: Baillière Tindall, 1990:759–79.
3   Brennan LJ. Modern day-case anaesthesia for children. *Br J Anaesth* 1999;83:91–103.
4   Moralee SJ, Murray JAM. Would day-case adult tonsillectomy be safe? *J Laryngol Otol* 1995;109:1166–7.
5   Gabalski EC, Mattucci KF, Moleski P. Ambulatory tonsillectomy and adenoidectomy. *Laryngoscope* 1996;106:77–80.
6   Cahill CJ. Basket cases and trolleys. Day surgery proposals for the Millennium. *J One-day Surg* 1999;9(1):11–12.
7   Cartwright DP. Death in the dental chair (editorial). *Anaesthesia* 1999;54:105–7.
8   Poswillo Report. Principal recommendations of the report. *Br Dent J* 1991;170:46–7.
9   Blayney MR, Malins AF, Cooper GM. Cardiac arrhythmias in children during outpatient general anaesthesia for dentistry: a prospective randomised trial. *Lancet* 1999;354:1864–6.
10 Bailie R, Barnett MB, Fraser JF. The Brain laryngeal mask. A comparative study with the nasal mask in paediatric dental outpatient anaesthesia. *Anaesthesia* 1991;46:358–60.
11 Hackmann T, Steward DJ, Sheps SB. Anemia in pediatric day-surgery patients: prevalence and detection. *Anesthesiology* 1991;75:27–31.
12 Malviya S, Swartz J, Lerman J. Are all preterm infants younger than 60 weeks postconceptual age at risk for postanesthetic apnea? *Anesthesiology* 1993;78:1076–81.
13 Welborn LG, Ramirez N, Oh TH *et al*. Postanesthetic apnea and periodic breathing in infants. *Anesthesiology* 1986;65:658–61.
14 Jacoby DB, Hirshman CA. General anesthesia in patients with viral respiratory infections: an unsound sleep? *Anesthesiology* 1991;74:969–72.
15 Tait AR, Pandit UA, Voepel-Lewis T, Munro HM, Malviya S. Use of the laryngeal mask airway in children with upper respiratory tract infections: a comparison with endotracheal intubation. *Anesth Analg* 1998;86:706–11.

16 Phillips S, Daborn AK, Hatch DJ. Preoperative fasting for paediatric anaesthesia. *Br J Anaesth* 1994;**73**:529–36.

17 Nicolson SC, Schreiner MS. Feed the babies (editorial). *Anesth Analg* 1994;**79**:407–9.

18 American Society of Anesthesiologists Task Force on Preoperative Fasting. Practice guidelines for preoperative fasting and the use of pharmacologic agents to reduce the risk of pulmonary aspiration: application to healthy patients undergoing elective procedures. *Anesthesiology* 1999;**90**:896–905.

19 Leigh JM, Walker J, Janaganathan P. Effect of preoperative anaesthetic visit on anxiety. *Br Med J* 1977;**2**:987–9.

20 Lawson RA, Smart NG, Gudgeon AC, Morton NS. Evaluation of an amethocaine gel preparation for percutaneous analgesia before venous cannulation in children. *Br J Anaesth* 1995;**75**:282–5.

21 Kain ZN, Mayes LC, Caramico LA *et al.* Parental presence during induction of anesthesia. A randomized controlled trial. *Anesthesiology* 1996;**84**:1060–7.

22 McEwen AW, Caldicott LD, Barker I. Parents in the anaesthetic room–parents' and anaesthetists' views. *Anaesthesia* 1994;**49**:987-90.

23 Black A, Sury MRJ, Hemington L, Howard R, Mackersie A, Hatch DJ. A comparison of the induction characteristics of sevoflurane and halothane in children. *Anaesthesia* 1996;**51**:539–42.

24 Sigston PE, Jenkins AMC, Jackson EA, Sury MR, Mackersie AM, Hatch DJ. Rapid inhalation induction in children: 8% sevoflurane compared with 5% halothane. *Br J Anaesth* 1997;**78**:362–5.

25 Sarner JB, Levine M, Davis PJ, Lerman J, Cook R, Motoyama EK. Clinical characteristics of sevoflurane in children. A comparison with halothane. *Anesthesiology* 1995;**82**:38–46.

26 Thwaites AJ, Edmends S, Tomlinson AA, Kendall JB, Smith I. A double-blind comparison of sevoflurane *vs* propofol and succinylcholine for tracheal intubation in children. *Br J Anaesth* 1999;**83**:410–14.

27 Townsend P, Stokes MA. Bradycardia during rapid inhalation induction with sevoflurane in children (letter). *Br J Anaesth* 1998;**80**:410.

28 Rieger A, Schröter G, Philippi W, Hass I, Eyrich K. A comparison of sevoflurane with halothane in outpatient adenotomy in children with mild upper respiratory tract infections. *J Clin Anesth* 1996;**8**:188–93.

29 Smith I, White PF, Nathanson M, Gouldson R. Propofol: an update on its clinical use. *Anesthesiology* 1994;**81**:1005–43.

30 Johnson RA, Harper NJN, Chadwick S, Vohra A. Pain on injection of propofol. Methods of alleviation. *Anaesthesia* 1990;**45**:439–42.

31 Welborn LG, Hannallah RS, Norden JM, Ruttimann UE, Callan CM. Comparison of emergence and recovery characteristics of sevoflurane, desflurane, and halothane in pediatric ambulatory patients. *Anesth Analg* 1996;**83**:917–20.

32 Lerman J, Davis PJ, Welborn LG *et al.* Induction, recovery, and safety characteristics of sevoflurane in children undergoing ambulatory surgery. *Anesthesiology* 1996;**84**:1332–40.

33 Hatch DJ. Propofol in paediatric intensive care (editorial). *Br J Anaesth* 1997;**79**:274–5.

34 Marsh B, White M, Morton N, Kenny GNC. Pharmacokinetic model driven infusion of propofol in children. *Br J Anaesth* 1991;**67**:41–8.

35 Reimer EJ, Montgomery CJ, Bevan JC, Merrick PM, Blackstock D, Popovic V. Propofol anaesthesia reduces early postoperative emesis after paediatric strabismus surgery. *Can J Anaesth* 1993;**40**:927–33.

36 Ved SA, Walden TL, Montana J *et al.* Vomiting and recovery after outpatient tonsillectomy and adenoidectomy in children. Comparison of four anesthetic techniques using nitrous oxide with halothane or propofol. *Anesthesiology* 1996;**85**:4–10.

37 Taguchi M, Watanabe S, Asakura N, Inomata S. End-tidal sevoflurane concentrations for laryngeal mask airway insertion and for tracheal intubation in children. *Anesthesiology* 1994;**81**:628–31.

38 Wilkins CJ, Cramp PGW, Staples J. Comparison of the anesthetic requirement for tolerance of laryngeal mask airway and endotracheal tube. *Anesth Analg* 1992;**75**:794–7.

39 Williams PJ, Bailey PM. Comparison of the reinforced laryngeal mask airway and tracheal intubation for adenotonsillectomy. *Br J Anaesth* 1993;**70**:30–3.

40   Quinn AC, Samaan A, McAteer EM, Moss E, Vucevic M. The reinforced laryngeal mask airway for dento-alveolar surgery. *Br J Anaesth* 1996;**77**:185–8.

41   Lopez-Gil M, Brimacombe J, Alvarez M. Safety and efficacy of the laryngeal mask airway. A prospective survey of 1400 children. *Anaesthesia* 1996;**51**:969–72.

42   Nunez J, Hughes J, Wareham K, Asai T. Timing of removal of the laryngeal mask airway. *Anaesthesia* 1998;**53**:126–30.

43   Varughese A, McCulloch D, Lewis M, Stokes M. Removal of the laryngeal mask airway (LMA) in children: awake or deep? (abstract) *Anesthesiology* 1994;**81**:A1321.

44   Robinson AL, Jerwood DC, Stokes MA. Routine suxamethonium in children. *Anaesthesia* 1996;**51**:874–8.

45   Rosenberg H, Gronert G. Intractable cardiac arrest in children given succinylcholine (letter). *Anesthesiology* 1992;**77**:1054.

46   Delphin E, Jackson D, Rothstein P. Use of succinylcholine during elective pediatric anesthesia should be reevaluated. *Anesth Analg* 1987;**66**:1190–2.

47   Steyn MP, Quinn AM, Gillespie JA, Miller DC, Best CJ, Morton NS. Tracheal intubation without neuromuscular block in children. *Br J Anaesth* 1994;**72**:403–6.

48   Yogendran S, Asokumar B, Cheng DCH, Chung F. A prospective randomized double-blind study of the effect of intravenous fluid therapy on adverse outcomes on outpatient surgery. *Anesth Analg* 1995;**80**:682–6.

49   Smith I, McCulloch DA. Anesthesia outside the operating room. In: White PF, ed. *Ambulatory anesthesia and surgery*. London: WB Saunders, 1996:220–32.

50   Morton NS. Prevention and control of pain in children. *Br J Anaesth* 1999;**83**:118–29.

51   Brown TCK, Eyres RL, McDougall RJ. Local and regional anaesthesia in children. *Br J Anaesth* 1999;**83**:65–77.

52   Cook B, Doyle E. The use of additives to local anaesthetic solutions for caudal epidural blockade. *Paed Anaesth* 1996;**6**:353–9.

53   Casey WF, Rice LJ, Hannallah RS, Broadman L, Norden JM, Guzzetta P. A comparison between bupivacaine instillation versus ilioinguinal/iliohypogastric nerve block for postoperative analgesia following inguinal herniorrhaphy in children. *Anesthesiology* 1990;**72**:637–9.

54   Tree-Trakarn T, Pirayavaraporn S. Postoperative pain relief for circumcision in children: comparison among morphine, nerve block, and topical analgesia. *Anesthesiology* 1985;**62**:519–22.

55   Watson DM. Topical amethocaine in strabismus surgery. *Anaesthesia* 1991;**46**:368–70.

56   Patel RI. Postoperative morbidity and discharge criteria. In: White PF, ed. *Ambulatory anesthesia and surgery*. London: WB Saunders, 1996:617–31.

57   Watcha MF, Simeon RM, White PF, Stevens JL. Effect of propofol on the incidence of postoperative vomiting after strabismus surgery in pediatric outpatients. *Anesthesiology* 1992;**75**:204–9.

58   Morton NS, Camu F, Dorman T *et al.* Ondansetron reduces nausea and vomiting after paediatric adenotonsillectomy. *Paed Anaesth* 1997;**7**:37–45.

59   Schreiner MS, Nicolson SC, Martin T, Whitney L. Should children drink before discharge from day surgery? *Anesthesiology* 1992;**76**:528–33.

60   Marshall SI, Chung F. Discharge criteria and complications after ambulatory surgery. *Anesth Analg* 1999;**88**:508–17.

61   Ræder JC, Korttila K. Regional anaesthesia for day surgery. In: Prys-Roberts C, Brown BRJ, eds. *International practice of anaesthesia*. Oxford: Butterworth-Heinemann, 1996:1–8.

62   Fisher QA, McComiskey CM, Hill JL *et al.* Postoperative voiding interval and duration of analgesia following peripheral or caudal nerve blocks in children. *Anesth Analg* 1993;**76**:173–7.

10: The future of day surgery

Ian Smith

Overview

This brief chapter will consider how day surgery may expand further in the future. The growth in day surgery has been rapid but not all areas or all countries have seen the same level of development. It is likely that some "catching up" will occur, so that patterns of activity become more similar. The ageing population will mean that day case patients inevitably become older and have more co-existing diseases. There may be changes in the day care process, with the adoption of some form of extended-stay facility for the more major procedures and a move into the office setting for the more minor cases.

In the past, developments in day surgery have taken place in parallel with the availability of a range of new drugs. More new general anaesthetic agents are unlikely, at least in the near future. Refinements to pain and antiemetic therapy are more likely and may have a significant impact on our practice.

Further developments in surgery are to be expected. Already, the growth of minimally invasive surgery has made some procedures possible on a day case basis for the first time. Further refinements may reduce the requirement for general anaesthesia and convert existing day case operations into minor procedures. The way in which some other conditions are treated may be altered altogether, establishing a completely new range of day case operations.

Introduction

Predicting the future is never easy. Looking back at the speculations of others often reveals that the pace of change was overestimated in many areas, while radical changes were missed altogether or their importance was not recognised. However, by observing what has happened in recent years while keeping an eye on developments which are already under way, it is possible to gain some insight into what is likely to happen in the next few years at least. Day surgery is an important topic in most developed countries and it is inevitable that financial pressures, aided by technological advances, will force its continued development.

The practice of day surgery

International variation

While day surgery has expanded considerably in recent years, this growth has been far from equal. The United States has been in the forefront of day surgery, followed closely by Canada, the United Kingdom, and Australia.[1] In these pioneering countries, 50–70% of all elective operations are day cases. Elsewhere, the picture is different. In the recent past, the contribution of day surgery was 30–40% in Scandinavia, less than 35% in Spain, 10–15% in Italy and even lower in Germany, several other European countries, much of Central America and Asia.[1] Even within a single country, there are considerable variations between different hospitals and regions.

The reasons for this variation are numerous. Day surgery may be under-developed because many patients live far from the hospital or because of safety concerns. More commonly, it is because the financial structure is such that hospitals, surgeons, and anaesthetists make more money from inpatient care. Until such financial disincentives are removed, day surgery will only be performed by true enthusiasts. Eventually, it is realised that day surgery substantially reduces the costs *per patient*, allowing more health care to be provided within a given time and budget. Spain, for example, has recently restructured its health management,[1] and day surgery is now expanding rapidly. Similar events have occurred in several Scandinavian countries. Once the economic conditions are right, "catching up" should be a rapid process, as there is now considerable experience to show which procedures, techniques, and patient groups are suitable and safe for day surgery.

Office-based practice

Day case surgery in the United States grew rapidly in the hospital setting. Subsequently, free-standing day surgery centres were developed and the move into the community has continued with office-based surgery. The practice of performing minor to intermediate surgical procedures in the surgeon's office is currently undergoing rapid expansion. Some operations are conducted with local anaesthesia only but in many cases sedation (monitored anaesthesia care) and even general anaesthesia are used. Office-based surgery is claimed to improve efficiency, make more effective use of the surgeon's time and provide a more pleasant experience for the patient.[2] In contrast, the less well-regulated and supported environment of an isolated office is seen as a major threat to patient safety.[3]

At present, office-based surgery is predominantly an American venture. Superficially, it appears to be a very economical form of health care and there is likely to be pressure for its adoption elsewhere.[4] Indeed, Spain is already developing office-based surgery,[2] and several other countries are considering it. The office must be considered a "hostile environment" and potential cases should be selected carefully to minimise the risk of perioperative complications. The facilities, equipment, and staff should be of a high standard, so that unforeseen eventualities can be managed as safely as possible. Emergency back-up will always be better in hospital, however, and this is a serious limitation of office-based practice.

If office-based surgery does spread in the future, we must be careful to learn from the lessons of the United States. There, the expansion of office-based practice outpaced regulation,[5] resulting in unsafe practices. For example, sedative and anaesthetic drugs were often administered by inadequately trained or improperly supervised personnel.[5] In order to avoid repetition of this disastrous situation, any development of office-based surgery should be preceded by appropriate safety measures and guidelines, preferably by modifying existing recommendations.[5-7] Britain's experience of office-based surgery has been mainly confined to dental practice. It is disappointing that deaths continue to occur [8] despite a number of expert reviews which produced many recommendations intended to improve safety. Rather than expand office-based surgery, there is currently a move to restrict the use of general anaesthesia outside the hospital environment.[9] Elsewhere, it remains to be seen whether office-based surgery will be so economical if all appropriate safety measures are implemented, certainly if general anaesthesia and sedation are to be used.

Extended care

Residual pain and postoperative nausea and vomiting (PONV) remain common reasons for unanticipated hospital admission following day surgery. The majority of these cases require only an overnight stay. In addition, a number of otherwise suitable patients are denied day surgery because they either live too far away or have nobody to look after them the first postoperative night. Both of these problems could be helped by some form of "extended care" facility. Day surgery generally implies that the patient is discharged home on the day of surgery but in the United States, it has often been defined as anything less than 24 hours in hospital. This broader definition allows more aggressive procedures to be managed as "day cases".

Laparoscopic cholecystectomy is a good example. Although some centres have been able to manage a high proportion of their patients as true day cases,[10] other workers have found a high same-day admission rate.[11] Even when patients are discharged successfully, significant levels of pain and PONV are common at home.[12,13] An overnight stay would improve the patient's experience and increase the detection of early postoperative complications.[14]

Extended care facilities may take several forms. Simply extending the hours during which a conventional day unit is staffed can allow more time for patients having extensive or late-starting operations to recover prior to discharge. Providing fully staffed 24-hour care will allow a far wider range of patients and procedures to be accommodated but is a relatively expensive option. Many patients will not require this level of supervision, however. All that may be needed is a basic "hotel" service. Some hospitals have developed their own facilities while others have made arrangements to use spare capacity in local hotels, with the patient being cared for by a friend or relative in the usual way. A more advanced design would provide a limited degree of supervision, coupled with the provision to administer parenteral pain and PONV therapy. It is likely that various types of extended care facilities will be developed further as the population ages and patients with more significant co-existing diseases are accepted for day surgery.

Drug developments

In the past, many of the developments in day surgery occurred in parallel with the availability of new general anaesthetic and adjuvant drugs. It is tempting to speculate that further developments will produce additional benefits in the future. At present, however, the likelihood of significant new anaesthetic agents seems rather remote. Several potential intravenous anaesthetics were abandoned because they offered no clear advantages or produced adverse effects. There are currently no new intravenous or volatile anaesthetic agents undergoing clinical trials. The inhaled anaesthetic xenon (see Chapter 3) is unlikely to be adopted because of cost and limited availability. Current anaesthetics are very safe and quite effective. Even if new drugs do appear in the next 5–10 years, they will have to offer very considerable advantages in order to justify their likely much higher cost. At the same time, existing drugs will lose their patent protection and their purchase cost is likely to fall.

In the absence of exciting new drugs, perhaps we will focus more on how to use existing drugs more effectively. Many believe that the way in which anaesthesia is performed is more important than which drugs are chosen. Improved forms of patient monitoring, such as bispectral index and auditory evoked potentials, may help us to better titrate our anaesthetic drugs in order to prevent overdose while still providing adequate anaesthesia. Computer-assisted (or target-controlled) drug infusions may make drug delivery easier and can make intravenous anaesthesia more accessible to the average practitioner.

Local anaesthesia

New local anaesthetic drugs have appeared recently (see Chapter 5). Both ropivacaine and levobupivacaine are apparently less toxic than bupivacaine and this must be an advantage. These new agents do not really alter the scope of regional anaesthesia, however. In the more distant future, formulation of bupivacaine in biodegradable microspheres may offer the potential of local anaesthesia lasting several days.[15] Such an agent would clearly be inappropriate for central nerve blocks, where motor and sympathetic block would also be prolonged. It might prove very worthwhile for infiltration anaesthesia or more localised nerve block, however, offering the prospect of prolonged and effective analgesia following more extensive surgery.

Adjuvant drugs

New and modified anaesthetic adjuvant drugs are possible in the future but radical developments seem unlikely. Fast-onset, short-duration non-depolarising neuromuscular blocking drugs like rapacuronium may supplement the muscle relaxant armamentarium but are unlikely to make new procedures possible. There was once much enthusiasm about α_2 agonists like dexmedetomidine, which produce an anaesthetic-sparing effect combined with analgesia and sedation. Unfortunately, prolonged sedation and bradycardia were found to be significant limitations.[16] However, dexmedetomidine is soon to become commercially available (as an intensive care sedative) and may yet find a place in day surgery.

Further 5-HT_3 antiemetics continue to appear. They may differ in cost, duration of effect, and side effect profile but do not appear to be any more effective than ondansetron. Neurokinin$_1$ antagonists are now under development, but it is too early to say whether these drugs will have a major impact on PONV. The use of antiemetics of different classes in combination is a logical approach which is only just beginning to be evaluated and may offer more hope for the future. In particular, the incorporation of steroids [17,18] into antiemetic regimens deserves further study.

Pain therapy

Pain remains a major factor limiting the expansion of day surgery. The goal of an opioid-like analgesia devoid of opioid side effects remains elusive, although some promising developments are occurring. Remifentanil allows adverse effects to be rapidly terminated, although the analgesic action is similarly short-lived. Other opioid variants, like tramadol, have not really solved the problem, as PONV remains problematic. Other classes of drugs will probably be necessary. In the distant future, peptide compounds have been isolated from sea snails which can produce profound analgesia without respiratory depression or nausea. Considerable development will be needed if these drugs are ever to be useful in day surgery.

At present, non-steroidal antiinflammatory drugs (NSAIDs) are important analgesics. Now that selective inhibitors of type 2 cyclooxygenase (COX-2) are available, the use of NSAIDs may be extended to some patients and circumstances where they are currently contraindicated. In addition, it has often been suggested that there is a ceiling effect to the efficacy of NSAIDs. It has been difficult to test this theory due to the occurrence of adverse effects at higher doses and it is possible that selective COX-2 inhibitors will permit larger doses to be given with a corresponding increase in efficacy. The combination of COX-2 inhibitors and extended-duration local anaesthetics (see above) may do much to improve postoperative pain management.

Surgical developments

Improvements in surgical techniques and the evolution of novel forms of operating are likely to profoundly influence the practice of day surgery in the future. Many examples of this can already be seen. In some cases, a development may remove the requirement for general anaesthesia and/or sedation. For example, flexible cystoscopy can be performed using topical local anaesthesia, whereas examination with a rigid instrument requires regional or general anaesthesia. Many diagnostic or follow-up cystoscopic examinations are now performed in the outpatient department or surgeon's office without the involvement of anaesthetists. Similarly, improvements in mammography and fine needle aspiration cytology have reduced the number of breast lumps which require excision biopsy.

In some cases, new surgical techniques are replacing traditional operations. One clear example is laparoscopic cholecystectomy which has largely replaced the open operation and made treatment of gallstones possible on a day case basis. In gynaecology, the diagnostic dilation and curettage was once extremely common. This operation has now been superseded by hysteroscopy and advances in instrument design mean that it is now frequently performed under local anaesthesia in the office. Laparoscopy may be moving in a similar direction. It is now possible to produce "microlaparoscopes" with an external diameter as little as 2 mm. These instruments can be inserted under local anaesthesia (supplemented with oral analgesia) and allow diagnostic procedures to be conducted with a minimum pneumoperitoneum on awake patients.[19] Laparoscopic sterilisation is also possible, requiring only light sedation.[19] At present, the optics of these small-diameter microlaparoscopes only permit diagnostic and "second-look" procedures, laparoscopic sterilisation, and assisted conception.[20] These are similar to the limitations of conventional laparoscopy only 20 years ago, however, and further developments in optical fibres may remove many more laparoscopic procedures from the current day case procedure list.

Other minimally invasive techniques are producing new potential day case operations. The use of a laser in place of conventional electrocautery can significantly reduce bleeding after prostatectomy and may permit same-day discharge without a urinary catheter.[21] Endometrial ablation is an effective alternative to hysterectomy for treating menorrhagia and may be performed on a day case basis.[22] Microsurgery to lumbar discs is gaining in popularity. Amazingly, awake craniotomy for tumour removal has been performed as a day case procedure,[23] although the majority of patients required a stay of one or more days. Minimally invasive cardiac surgery considerably reduces morbidity after coronary artery surgery; further progress could ultimately result in day case cardiac surgery. Minimally invasive repair of an aortic aneurysm through a small groin incision is already possible, although not yet a day case operation.

However, we must be careful to distinguish procedures which are *possible* in the hands of expert surgeons and specialist centres from those which can reasonably be adopted by the majority of day units. Neither must technology be allowed to develop for its own sake. A good example is laparoscopic repair of inguinal hernia. Unlike laparoscopic cholecystectomy, the open operation is already possible on a day case basis. Indeed, it may be performed using local anaesthesia, in contrast to the laparoscopic technique which requires general anaesthesia. Laparoscopic herniorrhaphy may be associated with more postoperative complications, delayed discharge, more severe pain in the early postoperative period and a greater likelihood of overnight admission compared to open repair under local anaesthesia.[24,25] Although there may be some benefits to patients following discharge, laparoscopic hernia repair has yet to match the very low complication rate of the open approach [26] and the long-term recurrence rate is still unknown.[27] This emphasises the need to evaluate all these new surgical developments critically before they are universally adopted.

Summary

The future will see further development of day surgery. There are clear economic benefits to day surgery and this form of health care is likely to be adopted by most countries as financial burdens increase. In the short term, much can be learned from those countries which already perform a significant proportion of their elective surgery on a day case basis. Development of day surgery beyond the levels conducted today may be possible with enhancements to aftercare of frail and elderly patients, those who live far from the day unit and perhaps those experiencing more severe pain and nausea. At the same time, more minor day case operations may move away from the hospital operating theatre and into the surgeon's office. This practice may reduce costs further but may increase risk unless adequate safety measures are put in place. Some would argue that anaesthesia in the office can never be as safe as in a hospital environment.

Drug developments have been important in the past and may continue to be so in the future. There is little immediate prospect of exciting new drugs but we may still have much to learn in the optimal use of existing preparations. Better management of pain and PONV are major priorities and several interesting new developments in analgesia offer some promise in the more distant future.

Refinements to surgical technique can significantly reduce postoperative pain and other complications, allowing operations which once required a prolonged admission to move into the day case setting, while other day case operations may be performed without anaesthesia at all. It is difficult to predict what new developments will take place in the future but from what is already under way, we can anticipate some exciting and challenging alterations to day case practice in the coming years.

1   White PF. Ambulatory anesthesia practices-an international perspective. *Sem Anesth* 1997;**16**:161–5.
2   R-Labajo AD. Office-based surgery and anesthesia. *Curr Opin Anesthesiol* 1998;**11**:615–21.
3   Gravenstein JS. Let no patient be harmed by anesthesia. *APSF Newsletter* 1999;**14**(4):44–6.
4   Ogg T. Office-based surgery: how should the International Association for Ambulatory Surgery proceed? (editorial). *Amb Surg* 1998;**6**:187–8.
5   Russell GB. Alternative-site anesthesia: guidelines affecting clinical care. *Curr Opin Anesthesiol* 1998;**11**:413–16.
6   Smith I. Office-based anaesthesia: the UK perspective. *Amb Surg* 1998;**6**:69–74.
7   American Society of Anesthesiologists. Guidelines for office-based anesthesia. *ASA Newsletter* 2000;**64**(1):16–20.
8   Cartwright DP. Death in the dental chair (editorial). *Anaesthesia* 1999;**54**:105–7.
9   Christie B. Scotland to ban general anaesthesia in dental surgeries. *Br Med J* 2000;**320**:598.
10 Voitk AJ. Outpatient cholecystectomy. *J Laparoendosc Surg* 1996;**6**:79–81.
11 Taylor E, Gaw F, Kennedy C. Outpatient laparoscopic cholecystectomy feasibility. *J Laparoendosc Surg* 1996;**6**:73–7.
12 Ræder JC, Mjåland O, Aasbø V, Grøgaard B, Buanes T. Desflurane versus propofol maintenance for outpatient laparoscopic cholecystectomy. *Acta Anaesthesiol Scand* 1998;**42**:106–10.
13 Singleton RJ, Rudkin GE, Osborne GA, Watkins DS, Williams JAR. Laparoscopic cholecystectomy as a day surgery procedure. *Anaesth Intens Care* 1996;**24**:231–6.
14 Saunders CJ, Leary BF, Wolfe BM. Is outpatient laparoscopic cholecystectomy wise? *Surg Endosc* 1995;**9**:1263–8.
15 Curley J, Castillo J, Hotz J et al. Prolonged regional nerve blockade. Injectible biodegradable bupivacaine/polyester microspheres. *Anesthesiology* 1996;**84**:1401–10.
16 Aho MS, Erkola OA, Scheinin H, Lehtinen A-M, Korttila KT. Effect of intravenously administered dexmedetomidine on pain after laparoscopic tubal ligation. *Anesth Analg* 1991;**73**:112–18.
17 Aasboe V, Ræder JC, Groegaard B. Betamethasone reduces postoperative pain and nausea after ambulatory surgery. *Anesth Analg* 1998;**87**:319–23.
18 Wang JJ, Ho ST, Liu HS, Ho CM. Prophylactic antiemetic effect of dexamethasone in women undergoing ambulatory laparoscopic surgery. *Br J Anaesth* 2000;**84**:459–62.

19 Phipps JH, Hassanien M, Miller R. Microlaparoscopy: diagnostic and sterilization without general anaesthesia. A safe, practical and cost-effective technique. *Gynae Endosc* 1996;**5**:223–4.

20 Daneshmand S, Surrey ES. Microlaparoscopy in the office setting. *Infertil Reprod Med Clin North Am* 1999;**10**:119–31.

21 Keoghane SR, Millar JM, Cranston DW. Is day-case prostatectomy feasible? *Br J Urol* 1995;**76**:600–3.

22 Goldrath MH. Hysteroscopic endometrial ablation. *Obst Gynecol Clin* 1995;**22**:559–72.

23 Blanshard HJ, Chung F, Manninen PH, Taylor MD, Bernestein M. Awake craniotomy for removal of intracranial tumour-a feasible technique for ambulatory patients (abstract). *Br J Anaesth* 1999;**82**(suppl 1):A28.

24 Rudkin GE, Maddern GJ. Peri-operative outcome for day-case laparoscopic and open inguinal hernia repair. *Anaesthesia* 1995;**50**:586–9.

25 Wellwood J, Sculpher MJ, Stoker D *et al.* Randomised controlled trial of laparoscopic *versus* open mesh repair for inguinal hernia: outcome and cost. *Br Med J* 1998;**317**:103–10.

26 Kark AE, Kurzer MN, Belsham PA, Neumayer L. Three thousand one hundred seventy-five primary inguinal hernia repairs: advantages of ambulatory open mesh repair using local anesthesia. *J Am Coll Surg* 1998;**186**:447–56.

27 Rose K, Wright D, McCollum C. Recurrence rate is true test of hernia repair (letter). *Br Med J* 1999;**318**:189.

243

Index

Page numbers in **bold** type refer to figures; those in *italics* refer to tables or boxed material